The Critics on THE INCURABLE WOUND:

THE
INCURABLE
WOUND

And Further Narratives of Medical Detection

BERTON ROUECHÉ

A BERKLEY MEDALLION BOOK
published by
BERKLEY PUBLISHING CORPORATION

To Lewis Thomas, M.D.

The contents of this book first appeared in
The New Yorker

Published by arrangement with
Little, Brown and Company .

BERKLEY EDITION, DECEMBER, 1958
2nd printing, November, 1960
3rd printing, March, 1963

BERKLEY MEDALLION EDITION, OCTOBER, 1964
2nd Printing, July, 1966

BERKLEY MEDALLION BOOKS are published by
BERKLEY PUBLISHING CORPORATION
15 East 26th Street, New York, N. Y. 10010

Berkley Medallion Books ® TM 757,375

Printed in the United States of America

Contents

Lost 7

The Incurable Wound 33

One of the Lucky Ones............. 58

$CH_3CO_2C_6H_4CO_2H$ 74

The Most Delicate Thing in the World 95

Ten Feet Tall 112

Lost

I'LL call him Uhlan—Walter Uhlan. The date was August 29, 1950, the day was a Tuesday, and the time was a little past noon. That, to the best of his subsequent recollection, was the moment of emergence. It was then that consciousness stirred and quickened, and he found himself—a tall, stooped, bespectacled man of thirty-nine, in a blue jersey and tan gabardine trousers, with a rumpled tweed jacket slung over his arm—standing in front of the Doubleday bookstore on the Long Island level of Pennsylvania Station. For several minutes, Uhlan had been cloudily aware of a mounting sense of strangeness and confusion. Now, with an almost jarring suddenness, he realized why. He didn't know who he was or where he was or what he was doing there.

Loss of memory is the familiar phenomenon familiarly known as amnesia. It invariably manifests itself as a disturbance in the essential processes that form the library of the mind. These include the prompt reception, the orderly conservation, and the accurate reproduction of mental impressions. Like those of most cerebral aberrations, its possible causes are almost astronomically numerous. All amnesias, however, stem from one or another of two distinctly different sources. They have their roots in either an organic or a functional debility. Of these, amnesia of organic origin is by far the more common. It is also less extensive, and less difficult to trace to its seat. The immediate cause of organic amnesia is a neural languor that renders the brain temporarily incapable of retaining and recalling stimuli. Organic amnesia is not in itself a disease, though, or even, in the usual sense, a symptom of one. It is merely a more or less insignificant corollary of some physiological dishevelment (an acute infection, an epileptic seizure, a metabolic convulsion) or an addling blow on the head.

The range of functional amnesia is protean (it may obscure little or much or even the whole of memory), its term is unpredictable (it may lift in a day, in a week, or only after many months). It is precipitated not by a mechanical breakdown but by the descent of an emotional block. Its gravest form, which science has come to call fugue, embraces three classically dramatic phases. The first of these is a brief interval of complete dissociation, closely resembling somnambulism. This is eventually followed by a period of lightened oblivion, in which only certain facts and events remain beyond the reach of the victim. The final stage, which may occur spontaneously or as a result of psychiatric manipulation, is a return to full-functioning consciousness. But, whatever its pattern, an attack of functional amnesia of the fugue type is seldom susceptible to either a ready or a reassuring explanation. In almost every instance, including, as it turned out, that of Walter Uhlan, it reflects the presence of a racking psychoneurosis—a constitutional inability to withstand the rigors of reality—whose beginnings lie deep in the encysted complex of the past.

Uhlan was an only child. He was born to Rufus Uhlan, a bookkeeper employed by a wholesale hardware company, and Grace Thompson Uhlan, the youngest of six daughters of a Manchester, New Hampshire, veterinary, in a railroad flat in South Boston on June 18, 1911. Ten months later, in the spring of 1912, Mrs. Uhlan developed acute leukemia, and in five or six weeks she was dead. During her illness, Walter had been taken in and cared for by his eldest maternal aunt, a childless widow with a comfortable pension, who lived just down the street. His mother's death prolonged his stay considerably. He remained there, cherished by his aunt and largely ignored by his father, until shortly after his fourth birthday. Rufus Uhlan had by then remarried and in July, 1915, having persuaded his bride to be a stepmother as well as a wife, he brought the boy home again. Walter endured a month of homesickness so keen that he still recalls it with anguish. Then, one afternoon, he slipped out of the flat, down the block, and into the arms of his aunt. After an hour of tears and kisses and cookies, she led him back up the street. That was his first attempt. By the time he was six, he had fled to his aunt at least a dozen times. Finally, a family council was called. Facts were faced, convenience was consulted, and eventually the problem was solved. Early in 1918, Uhlan was returned once more to his aunt. For several years, he spent every Sunday with his father, and they sometimes had an outing together. Then, as time went on, their meetings became less frequent. Toward the end of 1930, Rufus Uhlan was transferred by his firm to Chicago. The son never saw him again.

Uhlan was then nineteen. He had graduated from his neighborhood high school, he had passed a random year at Boston University, and he was restlessly in search of a job. He found one the following spring as a shipping clerk in the local retail branch of a mammoth mail-order house. It was the best he could do, and he made the best of it. In the course of the next ten years, he rose from clerk to salesman to assistant manager of the work-clothes department. But, with responsibility, his restlessness returned. After two years of executive tension, he resigned, talked things over with his aunt, and decided to study law. In the fall of 1941, he re-enrolled at Boston University. His second appearance on the campus lasted just six months. In February of 1942, his aunt suffered a coronary thrombosis, and he dropped out of school to take care of her. She died in the middle of May. Two months later, he was inducted into the Army.

Uhlan applied himself to the Army as he had to business, and with much the same result. At the end of the basic-training period, he was recognized as a potential officer and, because of his experience as a merchandiser, dispatched to the Quartermaster School at Camp Lee, Virginia. For the first ten weeks of a three-months course there, he was an apt and ardent pupil. Then an accident occurred. One afternoon, while he was demonstrating his ability to conduct close-order drill, a rumor reached him that a general recently returned from North Africa had joined the usual observers in the stand. Uhlan's reaction was sudden and shattering. He called out an order, tried to call it back, tried to give another, and then stood frozen with panic. His men shambled into a fence. Uhlan turned and ran from the field. An officer, investigating, discovered him a few minutes later, collapsed on his cot in an agony of tears. That was in February of 1943. The following October, after a regimen of rest and psychiatric rehabilitation at Walter Reed Army Hospital, in Washington, he was honorably separated from the service with a certificate-of-disability discharge.

Uhlan returned to civilian life in good health but low spirits. He had no plans, no prospects, and very little money. Also, now that his aunt was dead, he had no ties anywhere. During the next few months, he drifted from place to place—Philadelphia, Baltimore, New York —and from one aimless job to another. April found him back in Boston. There, one night in a bar on Scollay Square, he ran into a boyhood friend. It soon developed that he, too, was idle and restless and alone, and the two young men settled down to a long evening of beer and talk. They parted, toward morning, fired with a desire to go into business together. The notion survived a second meeting. All that remained was to turn up a promising project. By the first of June, they had one—a personnel service designed to supply wartime industry with competent maintenance men. It was a modest idea, but timely, and, to the best of their knowledge, unique. They opened an office, made the rounds of the local factories, and waited. The response was overwhelming. Before the year was out, they had satisfied clients from Maine to Maryland, and were scouring the countryside for recruits. But as time went on and the business steadied, Uhlan's enthusiasm waned. Finally, late in 1945, he was seized once more by the familiar longing for change. He sold out his interest, pocketed the proceeds, and began to drift again.

Uhlan chose, this time, to stay in Boston. The spell lasted almost a year. It ended, abruptly, at a cocktail party one afternoon in December of 1946. The reason was a girl. She lived in South Boston, where her father, a widower, kept a corner haberdashery shop; she had a job with an advertising agency on Tremont Street; and her name, I'll say, was Mildred Morris. Uhlan fell in love at a glance. His courtship was swift and triumphant. He and Miss Morris announced their engagement in February, 1947, and on the nineteenth of May they were married. Ten days later, after a honeymoon week in New York, at the St. Moritz Hotel, on Central Park South, they were comfortably settled in a pleasant apartment near Franklin Field. Meanwhile, inspired by love or necessity, Uhlan had ceased his drift from job to job and was again in business for himself. In March, he had conceived and set in motion a monogram-embroidering service. Like the employment agency, it got off to a most encouraging start. Throughout the spring of 1947, the orders poured in. Then, with summer, they began to dwindle. Uhlan told himself that it was merely a seasonal slump. But it wasn't. Fall was, if anything, worse. With the last of his savings, he managed to hold out

11

through Christmas. The creditors then closed in. Uhlan made his final appearance at his office on January 28, 1948. The following morning, he refused to get up. He said he couldn't. He said he had a paralyzing headache, he said he was a born failure, he burst into tears. A doctor, summoned by his frightened wife, arrived around noon and found him buried in the bedclothes, sobbing and moaning and shaking. Having taken his temperature and his history, the doctor gave him a sedative and suggested a consultation with a psychiatrist. He named a reliable colleague. Early in April, on the psychiatrist's recommendation, Uhlan was admitted to a suburban sanitarium for observation and treatment. Mrs. Uhlan went back to work and back to live with her father.

Uhlan's second immersion in psychotherapy lasted a little over six weeks. He was discharged, reasonably restored to normality, at the end of the third week in May. He returned to his wife, who continued to work, and a new apartment, and at once set out in search of a suitable job. He didn't immediately find one. The trouble was he didn't quite know what he wanted. His efforts were hampered by two contradictory desires. He was determined to somehow distinguish himself, but he lacked the nerve to risk another failure. He was still looking for an acceptable compromise when chance settled the problem for him. Shortly after Thanksgiving, his father-in-law was struck down by a hypertensive cardio-vascular stroke. It was neither fatal nor crippling, but it left him dangerously prostrated. What he needed, the family doctor reported, was several months of rest, preferably in a milder climate. Mrs. Uhlan did what she could. She gave up all thought of quitting her job, and arranged for her father to spend the winter with a cousin in Dover, Delaware. Meanwhile, she suggested, Uhlan could take over the haberdashery store. Uhlan heard her proposal with dismay. It was the mail-order house all over again, only worse. It was even more harrowing than the Army. It offered him responsibility, and no chance whatever to satisfy his ambition. But he couldn't very well refuse. Besides, it was only temporary. In the end, he reluctantly agreed to keep the business going.

In his new position, Uhlan opened the shop at nine in the morning. Five days a week, Monday through Friday, he locked up for the night at eight. On Saturdays, he stayed open until eleven. That had been Mr. Morris's custom. Uhlan was expected to follow it. During the first few weeks, in the intervals between customers, he kept busy by familiarizing himself with the stock. After that, in the intervals, he leaned on the counter and waited—for spring, for Mr. Morris, for his release. In June, Mrs. Uhlan had a letter from her father's doctor in Dover. Mr. Morris had suffered a mild relapse. It was advisable that he remain in Delaware through the summer. Uhlan took a deep breath. In September, the doctor wrote again. He felt it would still be risky for Mr. Morris to return to work. Perhaps a few more months of rest would put him back on his feet. Two weeks later, on October 7, 1949, there was another letter from Dover. Mr. Morris had just had a second stroke. There was, however, no particular cause for alarm. In fact, except for some difficulty in articulation and a partial paralysis of his left arm, he had made a strong recovery. But it would be understood, of course, that this new development meant that in all probability ... Uhlan put down the letter, and swallowed. He understood exactly what it meant. His stomach tightened with panic. He was trapped.

When Uhlan emerged to an awareness of his surroundings that August afternoon in 1950 and found himself lost and nameless in the depths of Pennsylvania Station, his first reaction again was one of panic. He stood for a moment transfixed. Then, as he moved on, an overhead sign caught his eye. It read, 8TH AVE. SUBWAY STRAIGHT AHEAD. His panic at once subsided. "I knew where I was."

13

he says. "Eighth Avenue and a subway could only mean New York. Well, New York was a place I knew. So I wasn't completely helpless. The next thing I remember was walking—and the heat. I've never been so hot. My shirt was soaking wet. Maybe I'd been running. I was on some street, and I had a vague kind of feeling that I was trying to get away from something. Or, rather, that I had got away. Because I didn't feel nervous or frightened, or anything like that. What I felt was relieved. Then I was looking at a telephone book. It was a classified directory, and I had it open to the section on hotels. I was tired and I wanted to take a bath and rest. The hotel I picked was in the West Forties, just off Broadway. At least, that was the one I tried first. But I only stayed a minute. The room they gave me was filthy. It had a ragged old rug on the floor and the bed was falling apart—that's my impression, anyway. I went down to the desk and asked for my money back. I didn't have any luggage, so I'd had to pay in advance. The clerk said no. I didn't argue. It didn't really matter. I just left, and went a couple of blocks up to the Taft. The room I got there must have been all right. At any rate, I took it. I remember looking at myself in the bathroom mirror. In a way, I guess, I was curious. All I remember, though, is thinking that whoever I was and wherever I came from, I hadn't been gone long. From the look of my beard, I had shaved that morning, and my pants were pressed and my shirt was reasonably clean. But, actually, I wasn't much interested. I was too tired. I flopped down on the bed and went to sleep."

Uhlan's deductions, as far as they went, were correct. He hadn't been gone very long. His wanderings had begun only that morning. "Walter left the house about eight," Mrs. Uhlan says. "That was a little early, but I wasn't surprised. We had agreed the night before that he would get breakfast on his way to the store. I was on vacation that week, and wanted to sleep late. Well, I heard him leave, and then I dozed off again, and it was after nine when I finally got up. Everything seemed perfectly normal. His shaving things were all over the bathroom, as usual, and I found his pajamas where I always did—on the floor beside the bed. I dressed and had breakfast and tidied up the house. Then I went down the street and did some marketing. When I got back, I thought it would be nice to call the store and say good morning. That must have been around ten-thirty. I called, but the phone just rang. There was no answer. I decided he'd probably stepped out for a mintue. Either that, or he was busy with a customer. I tried again at eleven. Again no answer. I waited a few minutes, and tried once more. Still no answer. Well, that *was* peculiar. I checked with the operator. There was nothing the matter with the phone. They just didn't answer, she said. But why? I'm not the nervous type, but I began to feel very uneasy. Something had happened. I was sure of it. It was nearly eleven-thirty by then. He couldn't be waiting on a customer for almost an hour. Or out. It wasn't possible. I tried to think what to do. Then I had an inspiration. I called the store next door. It was a little bakery, and the man who ran it was an old friend of Daddy's. I told him the story. He didn't know what to make of it, either. But he told me to hang on—he'd go take a look and see if there was anything wrong. He came back completely bewildered. Walter wasn't there. The front door was locked, the mail slot was full of letters, and the night light in the rear was still burning.

"I thanked him and hung up. I was too stunned to say another word. I was simply paralyzed. For a minute, I just sat there. The only thing I could think of was an accident. He was always in such a hurry. It always gave him the fidgets to have to wait for the light to change. I could almost see him darting across the street, and the brakes screaming, and the people running up—and the ambulance. But then I began to calm down. I told myself that you always imagine the worst. There was probably some perfectly ordinary explanation. Maybe he'd had to see one of the jobbers. Or our lawyer. There might even be some sort of trouble with the bank. He could have mentioned it the night before, and I could have just forgotten. That had happened more than once. So I tried to be sensible. I called the bank and the jobbers and the lawyer—everybody and every place I could think of. Even a few of his business friends. But none of them knew a thing. That left the hospitals and the police. I tried the hospitals first. I started with those near the stores. Then I called the big ones, like City Hospital and Massachusetts General. After that, I went straight down the list. It took me all afternoon, and I learned absolutely nothing. Except, of course, that he hadn't been hit by a car or suddenly taken sick. If he had, there would almost certainly have been some kind of record at one of the hospitals. At least, they'd have his name. Because his wallet was always stuffed with personal papers and all kinds of identification. I suppose that should have been some comfort, but it wasn't. I was frantic. In a way, I think, I'd almost hoped that a hospital would say yes. Nothing is worse than not knowing.

"My only hope then was the police. Even if they didn't know anything, they might at least be able to help. But I didn't have the strength to face them alone. I'd always been used to fending for myself, but somehow this was different. It was too much for me. I needed—well, moral support. So I called up a girl I knew and told her what had happened. If she wasn't my best friend then, she is now. She was simply wonderful. I couldn't have managed without her. She threw some things in a bag and jumped in her car and came straight over, and she stayed right through to the end. The first thing we did was drive to the store. I knew Walter wasn't there—I'd kept calling off and on all afternoon—but I wanted to see for myself. It looked the way it always does at night. I had a key, and we went in, and something made me open the cash register. It was empty. That meant Walter hadn't been in the store since he closed up the evening before. He never left money overnight at the store. He always brought it home with him. And he always put it back in the register the very first thing in the morning. It also meant that, whatever had happened, he was well supplied with money. He probably had over a hundred dollars. I looked around to make sure everything was all right, and then locked up again. Then we drove down to Police Head-quarters. We ended up in the Missing Persons Bureau. The sergeant there wasn't much impressed at first. When I told him that Walter had only been missing since morning, he gave me an awfully funny look. I think he thought that we'd quarreled or something, and Walter had simply walked out. But when he heard the whole story—about Walter's nervous breakdown, and so on—he couldn't have been nicer. Or more sympathetic. He said they'd send out a bulletin with a full description and recheck all the hospitals and do everything else that was possible. The minute they had some news, he would let me know."

It was a little past three when Uhlan flopped down on his bed in the Taft. He awakened at four, streaming with sweat but refreshed. Almost at once, a wave of restlessness rolled over him. It swept him off the bed and through the door and down the stairs to the street. "I had to get going," he says. "It didn't matter where. All I wanted was out. I felt hemmed in. Otherwise, though, I felt all right. And as soon as I started walking, I was fine. I completely relaxed. I cut over to Ninth Avenue, I remember, and headed south. I wasn't going anywhere and there wasn't any hurry. I just walked along looking in the windows and watching the people and enjoying the sights. It was an Italian neighborhood, and there were fruit and vege-table stands out in front of the stores. They were piled with wonderful food—all kinds of squash, and big yellow tomatoes, and a lot of things I'd never even seen before. I stopped at one place and bought a couple of beautiful bananas. Everything seemed new and different. Even the people. It was very interesting. But I kept on walking, and pretty soon I was in the Village. That was interesting, too. I was fascinated. I'd never been there before. There was one street of old-brick houses with shiny door-knobs and knockers, and I have a kind of memory of a bookstore window full of big pictures that looked carved out of wood. I don't really remember much about what I did, though. Mostly, I think, I just wandered around. I don't even know if I had any dinner. Maybe I had a ham-burger or something. I did have a few beers. But that was later on, after it got dark. It was still hot and I had a terrible thirst. When I couldn't stand it any longer, I'd find a bar and go in and drink a glass of beer. Then I'd start walking again. After one time, I remember sitting on a bench in Washington Square. I was smoking a cigarette, and it must have been late. It had that feel. The next thing I remember, I was back at the hotel.

"I hardly slept at all that night. It was too hot and I was too tired and I couldn't seem to get comfortable. Fi-nally, about seven-thirty, I stopped trying and got up. That was Wednesday morning. I took a shower and got dressed as fast as I could, and left. It was like the day before. I couldn't stay still. I had to keep moving. As long as I was going somewhere or doing something, I kept feel-ing all right. I must have headed straight for the Village. At any rate, I was back there by ten o'clock. My first recollection is one of those streets around Wanamaker's. There was a walk-up hotel in the middle of the block. I went in and got a room, but it was so dark and dirty I came right out. Then I tried another. It was even worse. I don't think it was even a real hotel. It was some kind of dive. The clerk asked me how many hours I planned to stay. So I walked out of that one, too. I kept walking until

I found a place that at least looked clean. It was on Eighth Street, I think, not far from Fifth Avenue. I sat in my room there for a while, just looking out the window. It was hot and sticky and beginning to rain. All of a sudden, I felt something crawling on my legs. It was a terrible feeling. I kicked off my pants and got under a good light and examined myself. My legs were alive with little animals. I don't know what they were. They weren't bedbugs or lice, or anything like that. I can't even describe them. They were sort of red and clammy and all tangled up in my hair—it was horrible. The only thing I could think to do was to shave my legs. I pulled on my pants and ran down to the street. There was a drugstore a couple of doors away. I went in and bought a razor and some blades and a tube of shaving cream. While I was at it, I bought a toothbrush. I felt filthy all over. Then I ran back to the hotel, and stripped, and got in the bathtub and started in. It took a long time. I really had to scrape to dig them out. They were practically embedded. By the time I got the last one off, my legs were bleeding in a dozen places. But I didn't care about that. The awful mess was down the drain, and I was clean. Then I scrubbed the razor and put in a new blade and had a regular shave, and brushed my teeth. Then I took a long hot bath. Then I got dressed and went out. I started walking again.

"I walked until it began to get dark. I don't know where I went. I was still in the Village, though, and so hungry my head was spinning. Except for a cup of coffee, I hadn't had a bite to eat all day. The part of the Village I was in was down below Washington Square. It was full of restaurants. The one I picked was an Italian place in a basement, with a menu in the window. I had a big plate of spaghetti and a bottle of beer. Then I felt better. After that, I walked back up to Eighth Street. I didn't have any plans, but when I came to a movie theater, I decided to go in. They were showing one of those Italian pictures—like *Paisan* or *Open City*. Also, I remember, there was a sort of lounge where they served coffee. I guess I saw about half the picture. But I couldn't get interested. I couldn't concentrate. Something kept kind of nagging at me. So I finally left and found a bar and had a beer. But that wasn't what I wanted, either. While I was standing there at the bar, it suddenly hit me that I didn't know who I was. I mean, it hit me in a new way. I'd been aware all along that there was something wrong, and every now and then I'd stop and wonder, but it hadn't really made any impression on me. This was different. I don't know how to explain it, but all of a sudden I was scared. It was as if I'd looked in a mirror and there wasn't any reflection. I remember standing there and trying to think. I thought of the hotel registers I'd signed, and tried to remember the name I'd written down. It was something Ward, I think, or Walsh. But I was sure that wasn't my name. It didn't sound right. I got to shaking so I could hardly hold my glass. Then I was out on the street, almost running. It was like something was chasing me. The next thing I remember, I was up in my hotel room. I started turning out my pockets. I knew I had a wallet. I remembered seeing it in the drugstore. If I could find it, there was sure to be something inside it that at least would give me a clue. But there wasn't any wallet. All I found was half a pack of cigarettes and some matches and money—all kinds of money. Every pocket was stuffed with bills. I don't know how much I had. I didn't count it. That didn't interest me. Instead, I took off my clothes and examined them. But they didn't tell me anything, either. My jersey had only an Arrow label, and all the label in my jacket said was Hart, Schaffner & Marx. Then I had an idea. I don't know how or why, but suddenly I decided I wanted to go to Philadelphia. I got dressed as fast as I could and ran down the street and headed for Penn Station. It must have been around three o'clock in the morning when I got there. Only I didn't go to Penn Station. I went to a bus depot near there. There was a bus just leaving, and I wasn't sure about the trains and I wanted to be in Philadelphia by morning. So I took the bus."

Uhlan arrived in Philadelphia, at the Broad Street Station, just after daybreak on Thursday, August 31. He found an all-night lunchroom near City Hall and had a bowl of cereal and a cup of coffee. After breakfast, he walked down Broad Street until he came to a hotel. "It was the John Bartram," he says. "They gave me a nice room, and I went to bed and slept for a couple of hours. I'd had a miserable night on the bus—hardly even dozed. When I woke up, it was gray and gloomy, and I felt terribly depressed. And bewildered. I didn't know what I was doing in Philadelphia. If I'd had a reason, it was gone now. I took a bath and got dressed. I needed a shave, but I'd lost my shaving things. Maybe I'd left them in New York, or on the bus. I didn't really care, though. I was too discouraged, and I was beginning to get jumpy and restless again. As soon as I got dressed, I went out and started walking. It was raining, but that didn't bother me, either. I walked the streets until I got tired. Then I went back to the hotel and tried to rest. After that, I walked some more. Every now and then, I had the feeling I was looking for something. I don't know what. Mostly, though, I just walked because I couldn't stay still. Pretty soon, it was dark. I was on Locust Street, I remember, carrying a little kit bag with a razor in it and some other things I'd bought, and I decided I'd had enough of Philadelphia. I had to get back to New York. So I walked over to Broad Street and up to the station and got a ticket on the next bus. I don't know when it left, but it must have been very late, because when I came out of the depot in New York, it was broad daylight.

"I had some breakfast in a cafeteria on Thirty-fourth Street. Then I headed back to the Village. It was another hot day, and something kept hurrying me, and by the time I got there I was dripping wet and half dead. The first place I went was that hotel on Eighth Street where I'd stayed before. But they were full up. Or so they said. Maybe it was the way I looked. I was filthy. I'd slept and sweated and walked through the rain in the same clothes for almost four days. Also, I had a two-day growth of beard. The only place that would take me in was a hole-in-the-wall down on Bleecker Street. Meanwhile, before I got there, I'd stopped and bought myself some underwear and a pair of socks and a regular shirt and a necktie. I still had the kit bag and the things I'd bought in Philadelphia. I showered and shaved and put on my new clothes. The old stuff I just threw in the wastebasket. Then I left. For a while, I felt better. At least I was clean. But then my mind started working. I got to worrying about who I was and what had happened. And what was going to happen. The only way I could keep halfway calm was to keep walking. Whenever I stopped, I'd begin to get panicky, and have to move on again. About two o'clock, I was in Times Square and I came to an out-of-town-newspaper stand. That gave me an idea. I was certain that I came from somewhere near New York. I had that feeling. And I was pretty sure it was a big city—because the traffic didn't bother me. That narrowed things down quite a bit. It was possible, I figured, if I got some papers from all the likeliest places, maybe one of them would look familiar. It might ring a bell. At any rate, it was worth trying. So I did. I bought a whole armful and carried them up Forty-second Street to Bryant Park and found a bench. I sat down and started reading. I began with Philadelphia—the *Bulletin* and the *Inquirer*. Then I went through the Baltimore *Sun* and *News-Post*, the Washington *Post* and *Times-Herald*, the Wilmington *News*, the Providence *Journal*, the Newark *News*, and the Hartford *Courant*. I ended up with the Pittsburgh *Post-Gazette*. But nothing happened. They all looked exactly the same. It was all I could do to keep from crying. It wasn't just disappointment. That was only part of it.

It was mainly—I don't know. I just felt so helpless, and alone.

"I don't remember leaving the park. The next thing I remember is some boys playing ball in a big field up on Riverside Drive. I sat on the grass and watched them for quite a while. Then I got restless, and started walking again. Around eight o'clock, I was back in the Village. I had a sandwich somewhere. It was a Greek place, I think. After that, I walked down to Bleecker Street. I realized that I'd left my kit bag in that hotel there and I had to get it. I couldn't afford to keep buying razors. My money was going too fast. By the time I found the hotel and got my bag, it was dark. It was hot, too, and I was thirsty. I walked around until I found a bar, and went in and had a beer. Only, it wasn't just a bar. It turned out to be some kind of night club. There was a band playing and people dancing, and pretty soon a floor show started up. One of the entertainers was a strip-tease girl. I stood at the bar and watched her. She wasn't pretty. As a matter of fact, she was kind of homely. But she had a beautiful body. It was really sensational. I guess she saw me watching her. When the show ended, she came over to the bar and said hello, and we started talking. I could hardly believe it. That was the first time in four days that anybody had even noticed me. It made me feel almost real. Her name was Arlene, she said, and then she asked me if I'd like to buy her a drink. That was the whole idea, of course, but I didn't mind. It was worth it. We sat down at a table and I ordered another beer and she asked for some whiskey. When the waiter left, she sat there for a minute, just looking at me. It was as if she hadn't really seen me before. Finally, she said, 'There's something wrong, isn't there? You're in some kind of trouble.' I was startled, but I told her no. I said I was fine. 'No,' she said. 'You're in trouble. I can tell.' Well, there didn't seem to be any point in arguing. So I told her. I told her the whole story—what there was to tell.

I don't know whether I expected her to believe me or not, but she did. She kept shaking her head, and saying, 'Oh, you poor thing.' She couldn't have been sweeter, or more understanding. She was wonderful. Then she jumped up and went over to the bar for a minute, and when the waiter brought our drinks, it was two beers. She'd canceled her whiskey. I had to save my money, she said.

"We sat there and talked until it was time for her next show. I waited, and after that we talked some more. She asked me all sorts of questions. She really tried to help. One question, I remember, was did I think I was married? I said yes. That hadn't really occurred to me before, but now I was sure of it. I had that feeling. Also, she wanted to know where I'd been staying. When I told her down on Bleecker Street, she threw up her hands. I ought to be in some place clean and decent, she thought. If I'd meet her when she got off work, she said, maybe I could get a room where she lived. That was a sort of apartment hotel up near Columbus Circle, and we agreed to meet there at around four. It must have been about one o'clock by then, but I'd had all the sitting and talking I could stand. I spent the next three hours just walking, and when I got to Arlene's place, she was in the lobby, waiting for me. But they didn't have any rooms. The clerk suggested the Alvin, on Fifty-second Street so we tried that, and I got a room there. Arlene handled everything. We sat in the lobby for a while and talked. Then we said good night. I think if I'd said the word, she would have come up to the room with me. She wanted to, I'm pretty sure. But I didn't. I couldn't. That was the last thing in the world I felt like. Not with anybody."

It was morning, on Saturday, when Uhlan fell asleep, but he was up and out by nine. After a cup of coffee at a drugstore, he walked down to the out-of-town-newspaper stand on Times Square. He bought another Baltimore *Sun* and, on an impulse, a Cleveland *Plain Dealer*, and then hurried back to the Alvin. The telephone was ringing as he let himself into his room. "It was Arlene," he says. "She wanted to know how I was. She also suggested that we have breakfast together. I didn't particularly want to—I felt more like reading—but I said all right. We met at a Childs, on Columbus Circle, and it turned out she had a plan. She thought I ought to see her doctor. He would know what to do. She gave me his address, and asked me to meet her there at three. I said all right to that, too. Maybe I meant it. But the minute I left her, I knew I wouldn't. Instead, I found a drugstore and bought a little bottle of toilet water and had it wrapped as a gift. I took it over to Arlene's place and left it, with a card thanking her for everything. I was grateful to her, but I'd had enough. She was beginning to make me uncomfortable.

"I bought some clean clothes and went back to the Alvin and changed. Then I took my kit bag and checked out. I'd been there long enough. I headed for the Village again. But it wasn't the way it had been. There were too many people and the streets were too narrow. Everything was different. I began to get panicky. That's the last thing I remember for I don't know how long. Then I was all alone on a path at the south end of Central Park, and across the street was the St. Moritz Hotel. I went over and walked past the entrance, and there was something about it. It meant something. When I reached the corner, I turned around and came back. There were people going in and out, and I stood there and watched them. I kept walking back and forth and hanging around the entrance and watching them for about an hour—until the doorman noticed me. He gave me a very suspicious look. I didn't want to leave. I hated to leave. There was something there that made me feel sort of sad and peaceful and almost happy. But I couldn't stay there with him watching me. I was afraid something might happen. The next time I reached the corner, I kept going. I kept on going until I came to a bus depot. It was around Times Square somewhere. There was a bus loading up. I asked where it was going and they said to Newark, and I don't know why, but I got on. It was something to do. One place was as good as another, I guess. We got to Newark at about eight-thirty in the evening. I found a bar and went in and had a beer. Then I walked around a little, and pretty soon I passed a burlesque house. That appealed to me. It sounded new and interesting. But it wasn't. The show was awful and the audience was worse. It was Saturday night, and everybody was drunk and yelling. I couldn't stand it. Besides, my feet were killing me. I left, and asked the ticket girl where I could find a decent hotel. She directed me to one called the Douglas. I got a room and went right to bed.

"It was too hot to sleep. Newark was even worse than Manhattan. I just lay there and looked at the ceiling and waited for it to get light. Finally, around seven, I got up. My feet were in terrible shape. They were so swollen I could hardly get my shoes on, and I had a big blister on my right heel. I squeezed into them, though, and got my things together and went downstairs. The coffee shop wasn't open yet. I sat in the lobby and looked at the Sunday papers and waited. When it opened, I went in and ordered a big breakfast—everything I could think of. My stomach was so empty it hurt. But when my order came, I couldn't eat. I was too tired and restless. After a few bites, I gave up. I had to get back to New York. It was as if I was missing something. They told me at the desk that the quickest way was the Hudson Tube. I guess I took it. I remember a tunnel and climbing a long flight of steps, and an empty street. It was almost ten o'clock in the morning, but it felt like the dead of night. It felt dark. There wasn't a soul in sight. There wasn't even a car or a truck going by. There was nothing but empty streets and closed doors and old warehouses. I felt like the last man on earth. There wasn't a sound, even— nothing. I didn't know which way to turn. Every street I tried looked just like all the rest. But I kept walking, and one of them came out at a ferry shed. It was the Erie ferry to New Jersey. I didn't want to take it, but I was afraid not to. I couldn't face those empty streets again. On the way over, I talked to a man and he told me I could get another Manhattan ferry on the Jersey side. It went to Christopher Street, he said. He even showed me the way. Maybe he was wrong. Either that or I didn't pay enough attention. Whatever happened, I never found it. The next thing I knew, I was in the middle of a railroad yard. There was nothing but tracks and freight cars as far as I could see. I started walking between two strings of cars. I walked for about a mile, and then the tracks ended at a high wire fence. On the other side of the fence were more cars. I tried to follow the fence, but there were old boxcars and piles of junk blocking the way, and I lost it. Then I was back in the middle of the yard again. I started climbing under the cars and over the couplings, trying to get out that way. But there wasn't any way out. I remember trying to run and I couldn't. I didn't have the strength. It began to rain. I crawled underneath a car and lay there. Then I heard somebody coming. It was a watchman. He saw me and started yelling, but I was already coming out. He was pretty tough for a minute. After I'd talked to him, though, he was all right. He led me down the tracks a few hundred yards to his shack. Beyond it was an open gate, and a street.

"I went out the gate and down the street, until I came to some buses. One of them was half full and ready to leave. I jumped on. That's the last thing I remember for about an hour. I must have gone right to sleep. When I woke up, it was the end of the line. I asked somebody where I was. North Bergen, he said. I looked around for another bus, and saw one marked BROADWAY. But it was the wrong Broadway. I ended up in Hoboken. I knew there was a ferry there, and I tried to find it. All I could find was bars. There was nothing but bars and drunks and hills. I tried to ask people the way, but I was too tired and groggy and miserable, and they wouldn't listen. They just walked on. Finally, it was raining so hard I couldn't keep going. I got on some bus. Then somebody was shaking me. I got up and got off, and I was back in North Bergen. I don't know how I ever got out of that place. I don't know whether I took a bus or a train or what. I don't remember anything more until I was standing on the corner of Forty-second Street and Seventh Avenue. That was about dusk. Then I was in Brooklyn, at the Hotel Pierrepont, on Pierrepont Street. I was sitting on a sofa in the lobby. There was a wedding reception going on in one of the banquet rooms. I could see the people talking and laughing. I sat there and watched them enjoying themselves, and I felt so lonely. It was worse than walking those empty streets. And all of a sudden I couldn't stand it. I broke down and started to cry.

"I woke up the next morning in a room at the Pierrepont. All my things were there—my bag, and my clothes, and a copy of *U. S. News & World Report* I'd bought—so it was my room. I must have checked in whenever it was I got there. I still felt groggy—everything seemed out of focus. It was as if I'd lost my glasses. And I hurt all over. It wasn't just my feet. Even my bones ached. Every move was agony, but I managed to get up and get dressed. I had to get out of there. I couldn't stay in Brooklyn. It was all wrong. I went down and checked out, and started up Pierrepont Street toward Borough Hall. It was close to eight by then, but the streets were deserted. There was hardly anybody even on Fulton Street. It didn't feel like Monday. Everything had that Sunday look. Then I realized it was Labor Day, and I don't know why, but an awful, helpless, terrified feeling came over me. I felt hunted. The only thing I could think of was to get back to Manhattan as quickly as possible. That meant the subway. I wandered around until I saw an entrance. It was the I.R.T., and I ran down the stairs and got on the first train that came along. But as soon as they closed the doors, I began to get uneasy. I was alone in the car, and I was afraid I'd made a mistake, and I couldn't stand it. Then the train stopped. I didn't know where I was, but I got off. I remember going up the stairs to the street. Only, it didn't seem like a street. There was a wall—a long, high wall. I started looking for a door or a gate or some other way out. There wasn't any. There was just the wall. I began to run. I ran as long as I could, and then I walked until I had to stop and rest. But the wall was still there. I started walking again. It was like a nightmare. I don't know how far I walked. It must have been miles. But finally I came to a saloon. It was on a corner in a block of factories. I went in and sat down and had a beer. The bartender was a big, smiling fellow, and I remember talking to him. He told me how to find the subway.

"I must have got off around Chatham Square. It was somewhere on the Bowery, anyway. The sidewalks were full of all kinds of bums and drunks, and there was an old woman lying in a doorway. She got up and came after me. I gave her a dime. It wasn't just to get rid of her. In a way, I knew how she felt. I knew how they all felt. The only difference was I still had some money. But I had to get out of there, too. So I started hurrying. At Houston Street, I cut over to Broadway, and then headed north again until I reached Times Square. After the Bowery, I felt dirty and contaminated, and I started looking for a hotel. I found one around three o'clock. It was the Century, on Forty-sixth Street, near the Luxor Baths. I showered and shaved, and rested a little. Then I soaked my feet in cold water so I could get my shoes back on, and went out. It was all I could do to walk, but I had to.

I don't know how to explain it. There was something driving me. It was getting closer and closer every minute, and I had to keep moving. I had to get somewhere. But everywhere I went was the wrong place. I remember walking down Madison Avenue, and how empty it was. Another time, I was way over east—around Beekman Place. Maybe that was earlier, though. Because I remember going through Union Square, and after that I was back in the Village, on Eighth Street. I didn't know which way to turn. Then I thought of the St. Moritz. I started back up Fifth Avenue. It was getting dark, and I tried to hurry, but I was too weak. I kept weaving and stumbling. Nothing had ever been more important. It was vital. I had to get there. But it didn't seem possible I could make it. I was too tired and sick and crippled—I'd never make it. It was too much, and I started to cry. There were people going by, but I didn't care. I couldn't help it. I couldn't stop.

"I don't know how I ever got to the St. Moritz. Or when—except that it was late. But I got there. I made it. I stood on the other side of Central Park South, where I could see the entrance, and watched. I kept looking at the faces of the women going in and out. It was as if there might be one I knew. I must have stood there a long time. Because finally I couldn't hold out any longer. I was too exhausted even to cry. I had to lie down. So I left and started back to my hotel. But I didn't know where to go. I'd forgotten the name of it, and where it was, and everything. There had been so many hotels. I turned back and went into the park. I sat down on a bench and tried to think. And I couldn't. My mind was dead. I was too miserable. It was cold and damp, and I began to get the shakes. Pretty soon, looking through the trees, I saw a policeman standing on the corner. I dragged myself off the bench and went over to him. He was very polite. I guess he thought I was drunk and was trying to humor me. At first, anyway. But after we'd talked a few minutes, I knew he believed me. He got interested. He suggested we go along to the precinct station on West Fifty-fourth Street. That scared me. I thought he was going to call the patrol wagon. I said I wouldn't be treated like a criminal. I said I'd go, but I wouldn't go that way. I pulled out a handful of money, and told him we'd go like respectable citizens. We'd take a cab."

Uhlan and the patrolman reached the Fifty-fourth Street station at about two o'clock in the morning. He told his story again, to the desk sergeant and to several detectives. They questioned him until nearly three. By that time, it was apparent that, whatever his trouble, he needed medical attention. He was taken first to St. Clare's Hospital, on West Fifty-first Street. The examining physician, noting that his symptoms were predominantly emotional, dispatched him promptly to Bellevue Hospital. There, after a crisp examination and a few questions, he was admitted for observation, and led away to bed in a psychiatric ward. "I spent an awful night," he says. "I'd heard about Bellevue, and when I realized that's where I was, all I wanted was out. I could hear people moaning and mumbling. I was terrified. But mostly I was in such pain. They'd almost had to cut my shoes to get them off, and my feet were like boils. They hurt so I hardly cared if I lived or died. Somehow, though, I fell asleep. Maybe they gave me something. I woke up crying, but there was a nice nurse standing there. She brought me some breakfast. She had a wonderful quiet voice, and after a while, I guess, I just lay there and rested. The next thing, the nurse was helping me down the hall, and I was in an office and a doctor was asking me questions. I tried to answer them, but my mind kept jumping around. I can't describe the way it felt. Then, suddenly, it was as if a door opened. All of a sudden, I knew. I remembered. I jumped up and shouted. I yelled, 'I know—I can remember! I remember my wife's name. It's Mildred. We live in Boston. I can even tell you the address. And my name is Uhlan—Walter Uhlan.' "

The Incurable Wound

ON October 30, 1951, a woman I'll call Mabel Tate, the wife of a West Texas cotton planter, was admitted to the Parkland City-County Hospital, in Dallas, with a tentative diagnosis of bulbar poliomyelitis. The record also noted, as is usual in ambiguous cases, two possible variant readings. They were epidemic encephalitis and, at the suggestion of the Tate family doctor, influenza. The general nature of her trouble, however, was somewhat less uncertain. All major signs and symptoms reflected a virus invasion, and one of massive, if not overwhelming, proportions. Mrs. Tate was blazing with fever, she was wildly agitated, and she was unable to speak, unable to swallow, and unable to move her left arm. Four days later, she sank into a coma, and died. Something about the manner of her death prompted the attending physician to request a clarifying post-mortem examination. The autopsy was done, with Mr. Tate's consent, early the following day. When the attending physician reached the hospital that morning, a report of the laboratory findings was on his desk. It began, "Encephalomyelitis with demonstrable Negri bodies in central motor neurons . . ." There was no need to read any further. That emphatically answered his question. Negri bodies are distinctive clusters of cellular substance whose presence in the brain has just one denotation. Mrs. Tate was a victim of rabies.

33

The attending physician once more sought out Mr. Tate. He told him what the pathologist had found and what the finding meant. That being the case, he went on to explain, two corollary conclusions were obvious. One was that Mrs. Tate had been attacked and bitten by a rabid animal. The other related to the approximate time of the attack. In view of the usual incubation period of rabies, he felt, it had probably taken place between two and six weeks earlier. The doctor spread his hands. All that remained was to establish the specific source of infection. It could have been a dog. It could have been a cat or a fox. It might even have been a skunk. There were numerous possibilities. Mr. Tate nodded. He appreciated the doctor's position. He doubted, though, if he could be of much help. It depended on what the doctor meant by an animal. His wife had been bitten, all right, and fairly recently, too. On October 9, to be exact. But it wasn't a dog or a cat or any of those. It was a bat. His wife had come across it lying in the road near their house. She had thought it was dead, and stooped down to take a look. The next thing she knew, it had jumped up and given her a nasty nip on the left arm. Then it had flown away.

The doctor hesitated. Very curious, he said. And certainly a most curious coincidence. He shrugged, and rose. But, of course, that was all it could be. The only species of bat in which rabies had ever been demonstrated was the vampire, and its range was limited to tropical Latin America. He was forced to conclude that Mr. Tate was mistaken. There must have been another animal episode. It could have happened as much as a year before. Such cases were uncommon but possible. Either Mr. Tate had forgotten or his wife had neglected to tell him. The doctor returned to his office and took out the record of the case. He closed it with the notation "Rabies, source unknown."

Officially, the animal responsible for the death of Mrs.

Tate is still not known. There is little possibility now that its identity will ever be irrefutably established. The rules of scientific evidence are too rigid for that. Nevertheless, in the opinion of most interested epidemiologists, the case no longer presents much of a riddle. Several subsequent events, they feel, have rendered it to all practical purposes clear. The first of these occurred on a cattle ranch some thirty miles southeast of Tampa, Florida, on June 23, 1953. Around ten o'clock that morning, the stockman's son, a boy of seven whom I'll name David Bonner, was playing in the back yard when a bat burst out of a nearby clump of trees. He called to his father, who was at work a short distance away, and pointed. Mr. Bonner glanced up, and stared. It was odd enough to see a bat abroad in the full light of day, but the creature's behavior was even stranger. The bat, when Mr. Bonner first caught sight of it, was circling the house. An instant later, it turned and streaked straight for the woods. Then it was back again—flying high, low, and every which way. Suddenly, from almost directly overhead, it swooped. David screamed, and tried to run. But it was too late. The bat was already upon him. Mr. Bonner crossed the yard in a bound. He caught his son and swung him about. The bat was clinging to the boy's chest, its teeth sunk deep in his flesh, and blood was staining his shirt. Mr. Bonner broke its grip with a backhand swipe. It dropped, with a strangled hiss, to the ground. He gave it a kick, for good measure. Then he picked up his son and carried him into the house.

David was more frightened than hurt. While Mrs. Bonner held and comforted him, his father examined the bite. It was an ugly wound but a small one, and not, Mr. Bonner decided, in any sense serious. There seemed no need to call a doctor. He cleaned the bite with soap and water, dusted it with sulfanilamide, and covered it with a gauze dressing. That—for the moment, at least—appeared to be sufficient. It didn't, however, put his mind altogether at rest. The circumstances of the assault, he had to admit, were, if nothing else, uncomfortably queer. Mrs. Bonner agreed. They held a hurried conference and reached a prompt decision. Mr. Bonner fetched his jacket and a paper bag, and returned to the back yard. The bat was lying where he had kicked it. Its fur was sandy brown, with yellow overtones, and except for its saucer ears and its long, web-fingered forearms, it might have been a field mouse. It was also, he was relieved to find, dead. He scooped it into the bag, and went on to the garage and his car. Forty minutes later, he was in the Tampa office of the Florida State Board of Health, closeted with a staff epidemiologist.

Mr. Bonner began the interview with a brief account of the incident. He then produced the bat and stated the reason for his visit. He wanted to have the creature examined. It was his understanding, he said, that bats were capable of transmitting rabies. He remembered reading in a livestock journal that they had been linked to an outbreak of the disease among cattle somewhere in South America. That was true, the doctor replied. There had, in fact, been many such cases, and not only among cattle. Several human cases were also on record. Bat rabies, as it was awkwardly called, was endemic in several Latin-American countries. They included Brazil (where the phenomenon was first reported), Honduras, Mexico, Colombia, Venezuela, Surinam, and the island of Trinidad. But, he pointed out, the bats involved were not ordinary bats. They were bats of a kind unknown outside the tropics. They were true, or bloodsucking, vampires. The bat that Mr. Bonner had brought with him was a harmless Florida yellow, a member of the species *Dasypterus floridanus*. It subsisted, like all other bats in the United States, exclusively on insects. Those were the facts. They didn't, of course, explain the attack. He had no theory about that. It was his opinion, though, that the facts held no cause for alarm. The doctor paused. However, he added, it was impossible to deny that the bat had behaved very strangely, and he quite understood how Mr. Bonner felt. A certain amount of uneasiness was only natural. Consequently, in order to settle the matter, he would send the bat along to the board's local laboratory for a routine brain examination. The result, he was confident, would be completely reassuring.

Mr. Bonner left the Board of Health at a little past one. By the time he reached home, it was almost two. At three, he was called to the telephone. It was the epidemiologist in Tampa, and he sounded stunned. He was calling, he said, from the laboratory. A bacteriologist there had just finished a microscopic examination of the bat's brain, and Mr. Bonner, incredibly, was right. The findings were positive for rabies. Arrangements were now being made for the usual confirmatory tests. They involved the inoculation of laboratory mice with bat-brain material, and would be done at the main State Board of Health laboratory, in Jacksonville. But that was largely a formality. The microscopic evidence was in every essential conclusive. Mr. Bonner's son had been bitten by a rabid animal, and it was imperative that preventive measures be taken at once. Could he bring the boy in to the Tampa office that afternoon? Mr. Bonner could, and did. The Pasteur treatment, as the immunizing procedure against rabies is called (in commemoration of its creator), requires a subcutaneous injection of antirabies vaccine every day for two weeks. David completed the course, apparently with success, on July 7, but because of the variable length of the incubation period in rabies, the summer was well over before it could be said that he was in all probability out of danger. That he had been in danger was beyond dispute by then. The Jacksonville tests had confirmed the fact, and so had an even more elaborate investigation, conducted at the request of the Florida authorities by the United States Public Health Service, at its Virus and Rickettsia Laboratory, in

Montgomery, Alabama. It was also certain by then that David's experience could not be dismissed as an isolated freak of misfortune. Late in September, while he was still under regular observation, a woman I'll call Frances Roberts suffered an almost identical attack, and that was closely followed by a third. The scene of both was eastern Pennsylvania.

The second Pennsylvania episode, though the least unequivocal of the three cases, was by far the most unsettling in its implications. Unlike the others, it happened in a city, and indoors—in a tavern in the central business section of Harrisburg. Its victim was a used-car salesman I'll identify as Carl Dayton. Shortly after midnight on Saturday, November 28, 1953, Mr. Dayton was standing with a group of friends at the tavern bar. Something brushed his face. He stumbled back, looked up, and saw a bat. It was dodging from wall to wall, just below the ceiling, and was heading toward the rear of the room. There was an open window there, but the bat made no attempt to escape. Instead, it circled back to the bar, lower now and moving fast. The bartender tried to whip it down with a towel, and one of the customers swung his hat at it. Both of them missed. Another struck out with a rolled newspaper, and caught it a staggering blow. It fell to the floor at Mr. Dayton's feet. He squatted down for a look, then sprang up with a yell and began to pound on the bar. His friends stood frozen, and stared. The bat was fixed to the back of his hand, and before he could shake it off, it had bitten his thumb to the bone. The bartender was the first to recover. He slammed the bat across the room, and this released the others. They charged the bat and stomped it to death and threw it into the street. That, to the impairment of the subsequent investigation, was the last of the bat. Then, more sensibly, they inspected Mr. Dayton's wound. It was obvious that he needed medical attention, and after bandaging his thumb with a handkerchief, they fetched a cab and sent him off to Harrisburg Polyclinic Hospital. From the hospital, where an interne (either unimpressed or unconvinced by his explanation of the accident) was satisfied to merely clean, close, and properly dress the wound, Mr. Dayton went home to bed.

Mr. Dayton, like David Bonner, is still alive, and for much the same reason. In his case, too, chance decisively intervened. Within an hour after the accident, a reporter on the Harrisburg *Patriot*, the city's morning newspaper, emerged from his offce, hailed a cab, and headed home. In the course of the trip, the driver began to talk. There was one thing about hacking, he said—anything could happen. Take tonight, for example. He had just come back from hauling a man to Polyclinic Hospital, and guess what was the matter with him. He'd been bitten on the thumb—by a bat! It was a mean-looking wound, too. His whole hand was covered with blood. But who ever heard of a bat attacking a man? He didn't know whether to believe it or not. Neither did the reporter, but it struck him that, if true, it was a possible story. The following day, on the way to work, he stopped by the hospital. A glance at the outpatient record established the facts of the matter. He then, with providential thoroughness, dropped around to the office of Ernest J. Witte, chief of the Division of Veterinary Public Health of the Pennsylvania Department of Health, and asked him what they meant. The case they described was news to Dr. Witte, but he answered without hesitation. They meant, he said, reaching for the telephone, that his division would investigate the incident at once. One phase of the inquiry would involve a search for the bat. Another, infinitely more urgent, would be concerned with Mr. Dayton. He must be found and returned to the hospital for immediate prophylactic treatment. The bat, in all probability, had been rabid.

Dr. Witte's hunch, though spontaneous, was anything

but blind. He had good reason to associate belligerent bats with rabies. The relationship, indeed, was one with which he happened to be peculiarly familiar. His knowledge derived not only from the alerting example of the Bonner episode, a bulletin on which the Public Health Service had promptly dispatched to all state health officers, but also, more recently, from direct professional experience. That had been provided by the case of Frances Roberts. On the afternoon of September 29, as Dr. Witte later reported to the American Public Health Association, Mrs. Roberts, the wife of an amateur ornithologist of Boiling Springs, an upland resort about twenty miles west of Harrisburg, had accompanied her husband on a canoeing jaunt across a lake near their home. Toward six o'clock, deciding to stretch their legs before turning back, they beached their craft on a wooded shore, and Mr. Roberts wandered off to observe a flock of waterfowl.

Mrs. Roberts stayed by the canoe, and she was standing there, Dr. Witte noted in his report, when "a bat suddenly landed on [her] upper arm, and bit her without warning or provocation. The woman . . . was startled by the attack and could not immediately identify the object clinging to her arm. Because of her fright, she does not recall distinct biting sensations, although she was conscious of the creature's scratching. Still not knowing what the object was, she finally grabbed the bat with her other hand and threw it against a nearby fence, where it remained stunned by the blow. [Mr. Roberts] was attracted by the commotion and quickly identified the animal as a [hoary, or *Lasiurus cinereus*] bat. Being a naturalist, with considerable knowledge and background in wildlife, he quickly recognized the behavior of the bat to be abnormal. He had the presence of mind to act with swiftness and cleverly trapped the creature in a pail, which he had nearby, and covered it with a newspaper. In a matter of minutes, the party headed back by canoe

. . . to their home. [Mrs. Roberts] proceeded immediately to the doctor for treatment. . . . The physician reported that the patient received attention within one hour after the biting episode. He scrubbed the wound thoroughly with surgical soap and cauterized the wound, using an electric cautery. There were three distinct tooth marks on the upper arm, between the elbow and shoulder. He then called the [State] Health Department for advice on the handling of this case. Motivated to a large degree by the reports of the Florida experience, we immediately recommended antirabies prophylaxis." At the same time, Mr. Roberts was asked to deliver the bat to the Harrisburg laboratory of the department's Bureau of Animal Industry. He did so the following morning. "Touch preparations and, later, sections of the bat's brain revealed typical Negri bodies," Dr. Witte continued. "These were confirmed by the Director of Laboratories, Pennsylvania Department of Health, and by the Virus and Rickettsia Laboratory of the U. S. Public Health Service. Two rabbits were injected intracranially with the bat-brain material. Both animals developed clinical symptoms of rabies and died [within] twenty-seven days. [Meanwhile], starting October 1, [Mrs. Roberts] received fourteen injections of vaccine. [She] suffered no adverse reactions during the entire course of treatment. . . . As of this date [November 10, 1953], she remains in good health, but is still under her physician's care."

Although it was Dr. Witte who brought the attack on Mrs. Roberts to general medical attention, his report was not the first account of her misadventure. The first was a newspaper story, less conprehensive but equally stirring, that was widely published throughout the East within a day or two of the incident. Among those whom it particularly stirred was Frederick R. Taylor, an internist and professor of medical literature at the Bowman Gray School of Medicine of Wake Forest College, in Wake

Forest, North Carolina. The news did not merely startle Dr. Taylor. It also inspired him to reflection, the nature of which he presently communicated to a colleague in Georgia. His letter, which has been preserved, began with a forceful summary of the Roberts case. This was followed by some lines to the effect that he had long been imperturbably aware of the existence of rabies in Latin-American vampires. "But," he then exclaimed, "an ordinary, insectivorous bat!!! What would happen if the Western bats that live literally by the millions in Carlsbad Caverns, New Mexico, got an epidemic started there? I have seen a high cloud of countless hordes of bats come out of the caverns' mouth at dusk. Too horrible to contemplate!"

Dr. Taylor's letter was dated October 19, 1953. Little more than two years later, on February 1, 1956, a news story authorized by the New Mexico State Department of Public Health appeared in the Santa Fe *New Mexican* under a six-column headline reading, "CARLSBAD CAVE BATS INFECTED WITH RABIES." "Rabies," it began, "has been discovered among the millions of bats at Carlsbad Caverns. It was a rabies epidemic which caused the death of hundreds of the Caverns bats in August and September of last year." The account continued:

Last Aug. 20, officials of the National Park Service at Carlsbad noticed dead and dying bats in increasing numbers. They were found on the floor of the caverns and in its entrance. Ranchers in the area also found dead bats. At that time it was thought that extensive insecticide spraying might have caused the deaths during the 10-day epidemic. But tests by the U. S. Public Health Service found no evidence of this. Instead, tests were begun to see if rabies had caused the deaths.

Lt. Col. Kennet Burns, chief of the veterinary virus laboratory at Ft. Sam Houston, Tex., collected specimens of dead and dying bats for examination while the epidemic was going on. Virus examinations by Burns revealed the presence of rabies in more than 50 per cent of the specimens, the department said. In addition, blood samples from a large number of live bats collected in flight at the caverns after the epidemic showed the presence of antibodies against rabies, indicating that many of the bats had been exposed to the disease some time in the past. . . .

The story also stated that although no human being had ever been known to be bitten by a bat while visiting the caverns, the health authorities had warned people against touching any of the creatures they might find dead or dying there.

Rabies is one of around sixty human diseases now known, or confidently supposed, to be of viral origin. Its causative agent is thus a member of the most mysterious form of life on earth. About all that can be said of the viruses is that they are supremely small (some are only just within the reach of an electron microscope), infinitely numerous (not even the bacteria are more ubiquitous) and almost incomparably specialized. All viruses are obligate intracellular parasites. They share with the rickettsiae the otherwise unique distinction of being unable to grow or reproduce outside the protoplasmic tissue of a living host. In general, the severity of a viral invasion reflects the functional importance of the particular cells to which the invaders are drawn. The virus of rabies is a neurotropic virus. Like the viruses of poliomyelitis and the several encephalitides, it has a special affinity for the cells of the central nervous system. It has, however, little else in common with any other virus. Its range, for one thing, is extraordinarily wide. Unlike the great majority of viruses (including the agents of smallpox, measles, yellow fever, poliomyelitis, infectious hepatitis, and the common cold), which can find in nature fewer than half a dozen satisfactory habitats, it is able to exist comfortably and abundantly proliferate in any warm-blooded animal. Its means of transmission is also peculiarly its own. Most viruses insinuate themselves into a host through either the respiratory passage or the gastrointestinal tract. A few are conveyed by bloodsucking insects. The rabies virus enters by way of a bite contaminated with the saliva of one of its victims. In this respect, it might seem to resemble the various mosquito-borne viruses, but the resemblance is merely apparent. The latter are transmitted in the natural course of the carrier's search for food. There is nothing natural about the transfer of the rabies virus. It wrings collaboration from its carrier hosts by torturing them into a homicidal fury. The incubation period of rabies (or the interval between the implantation of the organism and its establishment in the brain) is largely determined by the depth of the wound, its proximity to the brain, and the size of the original viral colony. This period, though disconcertingly variable, is seldom shorter than fifteen days and almost never longer than a year. But whether the virus reaches its destination in days or weeks or months, the result is inevitably the same. Rabies, in man, is a fatal disease. No recoveries are known.

The symptomatology of rabies is essentially the same in all susceptible animals. There are only superficial differences. The onset of the disease is generally mild and always indistinct. In man (and, insofar as can be determined, most comparably complicated animals), its earliest manifestations are those of any infection—a little fever, a dull headache, a scratchy throat, occasional nausea. This phase frequently lasts for two or three days, and sometimes even four, and is followed by a tingling pain at the site of the wound—the first diagnostically significant indication of rabies. Its grip, already fixed beyond release, then suddenly tightens. The muscles stiffen, the nerves tense, and the mind begins to fray with temper and apprehension. Anxiety quickens into fear. There is a vivid sense of approaching doom, a certainty of death. "A [rabid] patient weighed down with terror often becomes maniacal," D. L. Harris, medical director of the Pasteur Clinic in St. Louis, noted in a recent clinical study. "An excessive flow of thick tenacious saliva pours over his face and neck and becomes smeared on his hands and clothes and over the bedding and floor. These periods of rage are followed by moments of calm in which [he] usually shows anxiety for the safety of those around him and warns them of the approach of another crisis. Hyperesthesia of the skin to changes of temperature, and especially to currents of air, and increased sensitiveness to sound and light mark the progress of cerebral irritation. Convulsions are brought on by the least irritation and by the slightest current of air . . . the breath comes in spasms, dyspnea is extreme, and there are epileptiform seizures or titanic rigidity. Hydrophobia is rarely absent . . . When the patient [attempts to drink], there is an immediate viselike contraction of the muscles of deglutition with an excruciatingly painful spasm of the glottis and the pharynx. The body trembles with convulsive movements, the jaws are clenched, respiration is impossible. . . . After several attempts to drink, the pain is so terrible that despite intense thirst [the patient] cannot be induced to try to swallow liquids, and the sight of water or mention of the word brings on an attack. As a rule, death occurs after two or three days from cardiac or respiratory failure."

Although all highly developed animals are equally responsive to its gothic embrace, the rabies virus has its favored circle of hosts. It is naturally most inclined to frequent those best equipped to further its spread. This largely confines its normal range to the more prolific and short-tempered carnivores, a group that includes the fox, the wolf, the coyote, the jackal, the skunk, the mongoose, the cat, and the dog. Of these, the last, for reasons still obscure, has always been its most consistently conspicuous victim. The dog is also the animal in which its depredations were first recognized as those of a specific disease. Just when that occurred is uncertain. An illusion in the *Iliad* to "canine madness" has persuaded many medical historians that rabies may have been known to the Mediterranean world as early as the tenth century before Christ, and most believe, on the basis of rather stronger internal evidence, that the fifth-century Greek philosopher Democritus, who is chiefly remembered as a pioneer atomic theoretician and the teacher of Hippocrates, was probably conscious of its existence. The first explicit reference to rabies of which there is any record was set down by Aristotle, around 335 B.C., in his *Historia Animalium*. "Dogs suffer from three diseases: lyssa, quinsy, and sore feet," he noted. "Lyssa drives the animal mad, and any animal whatever, excepting man, will take the disease if bitten by a dog so afflicted; the disease is fatal to the dog itself, and to any animal it may bite, man excepted." Lyssa, a transliteration of *Aʹvooa*, means "frenzy," and is the name by which rabies was originally known. The Romans gave the disease its modern name, which derives from *rabere*, the Latin for "to rage," and has been in common usage since the first Christian century.

The Romans also modernized the Greek conception of rabies. A gifted encyclopedist of the early empire named Aulus Cornelius Celsus was among the first to raise his eyes from the pages of *Historia Animalium* and look squarely at the world around him. Having done so, he proceeded to challenge the first of Aristotle's comfortable exceptions as myopically veterinarian. All animals, he decided in his classic *De Medicina*, were equally susceptible to rabies. Celsus was willing, however, to concede Aristotle's second exception. It was possible, his studies informed him, that the disease could be mastered in man. He then went on to propose a still valid preventive technique ("the wound . . . must be cauterized") and, less acutely, an antidote and a course of treatment. This consisted of thirty herbal ingredients (including poppy tears, Illyrian iris, Gallic nard, white pepper, male frankincense, and turpentine) mixed with honey and dissolved in a tumbler of wine. Its omission, he added, was risky. "When too little has been done for such a wound it usually gives rise to a fear of water," he wrote. "In these cases there is very little hope for the sufferer. But still there is just one remedy, to throw the patient unawares into a water tank which he has not seen beforehand. If he cannot swim, let him sink under and drink, then lift him out. If he can swim, push him under at intervals so that he drinks his fill of water even against his will. For so his thirst and dread of water are removed at the same time. Yet this procedure incurs a further danger, that a spasm of sinews, provoked by the cold water, may carry off a weakened body. Lest this should happen, he must be taken straight from the tank and plunged into a bath of hot oil."

Celsus's uneasy concession that rabies need not be fatal to man was accepted without recorded dispute for fifteen hundred years. So, except for certain pharmacological refinements, were his methods of breaking its hold. Pedanius Dioscorides, whose *De Materia Medica* was the standard pharmacopoeia throughout the Roman era, contented himself with offering two alternative antidotes. One was a draught of hippocampus, or sea-horse, ashes. The other had as its active principle the leaves of the bladder campion. "This, being beaten when it is green, with old swine's grease, is good for the mad-dog-bitten," he wrote. Rufus of Ephesus, a second-century physiologist, preferred a draught of "wormwood, aristolochia, Lycian thorn, decoction of river-crayfish, water-germander, rock-parsley, and the root called gentian." Even Galen, the most observant, as well as the most imaginative, medical investigator in the millennia between Hippocrates and the Renaissance, had nothing to add to Celsus but a polished definition: "[Rabies] is a disease that follows the bite of a mad dog and is accompanied by an aversion to drinking liquids, convulsions, and hiccups. Sometimes maniacal attacks supervene."

After Galen, and the subsequent canonization of Greco-Roman medicine, the illumination of rabies, like that of all disease, was considered complete, and the subject complacently closed. The first attempt to reopen it was made in the sixteenth century. A Veronese savant named Hieronymus Fracastorius is usually celebrated for this act of desecration. Rabies, he announced in 1546, in his precocious *Contagions, and Contagious Diseases and Their Treatment*, was an infectious disease, always communicated by the injection of saliva into the blood, and, not-withstanding the protestations of pharmacy, always irremediably fatal. He also emphasized this novel conception of the disease in a dissertation on hunting dogs. "What particularly calls for the care of the skilled mind," he wrote, "is when, inflamed with rabies, [the dog] attacks now these, now those and, turning against the master himself, he inflicts the incurable wound." Fracastorius was a man of towering intellectual stature. In addition to being a notable physician, he was a poet (the term "syphilis" derives from his *A Poetical History of the French Disease*), a botanist, a geographer, a musician, a mathematician, and an astronomer, and his morbid view of rabies received a respectful hearing. It even, for a time, attracted a few admirers. But hope and habit were too strong, and within a generation the more congenial classic conception resumed its interrupted vogue.

Celsus's hydrotherapeutic regimen, adapted to the ducking stool, was commonly prescribed in cases of rabies throughout the sixteenth and seventeenth centuries, and at least on occasion (an essay by Oliver Goldsmith, written around 1765, refers to "a little boy bit in the leg, and gone down to be dipped in the salt water") during much of the eighteenth century. His pharmacological influence continued even longer. In 1806, the New York State Legislature passed, without recorded opposition, a bill entitled "An Act for Granting a Compensation to John M. Crous, for Discovering and Publishing a Cure for the Canine Madness." Crous's cure, for which he was granted a thousand dollars, was a tablet to be swallowed with water. Its components included the pulverized jawbone of a dog, the dried false tongue of a newly foaled colt, and a pinch of corroded copper taken from an English penny minted in the reign of George I. Other American physicians of that time, perhaps less impressed by royalty, favored a remedy composed of bole armeniac, alum, chalk, elecampane, and black pepper. They also had confidence, as did many European doctors, in the curative powers of concretions, similar to kidney stones, that are sometimes found in the intestines of deer, goats, and other herbivorous animals and that, because they were used as a specific in the treatment of rabies, became known as madstones. Such concretions, being formed of mineral salts, are porous and somewhat absorbent. These qualities helped to support the belief that a madstone applied to a rabic wound would promptly extract the venom. "This afternoon called on by a man in Jeffersonville to apply the madstone to a little son bitten a day or two previous," an Indiana judge, soldier, and statesman named John McCoy noted in his journal on June 9, 1848. "Rode thro' the rain and reached there about sunset. Induced to think the dog mad." In 1879, at an auction in Texas a madstone brought two hundred and fifty dollars. That would be the equivalent of about a thousand dollars today.

The supposition that rabies could be cured by some curious pill or poultice expired with the nineteenth century. The absolute lethality of the disease is now universally accepted. One reason for this abrupt resignation to reality is that the evidence assembled by modern medical science leaves no room for doubt. Another is that the truth is no longer unbearable. Since the eighteen-eighties, when Pasteur was inspired to adapt to rabies his epochal discovery that the pathogenic properties of a microorganism can be attenuated (by drying, or treatment with certain chemicals, and passage through a succession of laboratory animals) without affecting its capacity to generate protective antibodies, a reliable means of hobbling the disease has been everywhere at hand.

Pasteur conceived the idea of rabies prophylaxis in 1880. By the end of 1883, he and his associates at the Ecole Normale, in Paris, were able to produce a stable strain of suitably domesticated virus. This was followed by two series of experiments establishing beyond dispute that the strain was immunologically effective in dogs. The first of these was brought to a brilliant close in June, 1884, with a formal trial before a committee of scientists appointed by the French Government. For this definitive test, Pasteur chose two previously vaccinated dogs, two untreated dogs, and two untreated rabbits. After being examined by the committee, the six animals were anesthetized and trephined. Each animal was then identically inoculated with a quantity of material drawn from the brain of a demonstrably rabid dog. When the operation was completed, the animals were separately confined, and all received the same postoperative care. Two weeks later, the four controls, or untreated animals, developed rabies, and died. The vaccinated dogs remained in normal health. The second series of experiments, though begun at about the same time, continued into the following year, and the results were equally emphatic. They showed that it was possible to immunize a dog against rabies not only before but, if the step was undertaken promptly, after exposure to the disease. Pasteur emerged from this revolutionary triumph with a vision of one even more revolutionary. "What I aspire to [now] is the possibility of treating a man after a bite with no fear of accidents," he wrote in the spring of 1885. ". . . I have not yet dared to treat human beings after bites from rabid dogs. But the time is not far off."

The time, as it turned out, was only a few weeks off. Pasteur treated his first human patient on July 6, 1885. This now famous pioneer was a nine-year-old Alsatian boy named Joseph Meister. Two days before, while walking on a country road near his home, he had been attacked by a plainly rabid dog, knocked down, and bitten fourteen times. When Pasteur saw him, at the request of a family doctor, the boy was more dead than alive. In fact, Pasteur later recalled, it was only the apparent hopelessness of the case that induced him to attempt its treatment. The procedure he used was a freehand adaptation of the one he had developed in his most recent experiments with dogs, and it took ten days. During that time, the boy received thirteen inoculations, of increasingly potent vaccine. His immediate reaction was encouraging, and it continued satisfactory throughout the treatment. At the end of a month, his wounds having healed, he seemed to be fully recovered. He was. Joseph Meister lived to be sixty-four. He died in 1940, a suicide.

The rehabilitation of Joseph Meister, which Pasteur described in a paper entitled "Méthode pour Prévenir la Rage après Morsure" and presented at a meeting of the Académie des Sciences on October 26, 1885, created an instant and appreciative stir throughout the medical world. "[Rabies], that dread disease against which all therapeutic measures had hitherto failed, has at last found a remedy," the formidable neuropathologist Edmé-Félix-Alfred Vulpian proclaimed. Assisted by this and other resounding testimonials, the Pasteur treatment, as the procedure came to be called, was in international use within a decade, and it has since been administered many thousands of times, with sufficient success to establish its worth as a reliable defensive tool. Or so it is generally assumed. To what extent the Pasteur treatment protects human beings against the development of rabies, however, is not known, and probably (in view of the natural scarcity of volunteers available for a series of controlled experiments) never will be. Its powers, in any event, are somewhat less than total. In a recent monograph, Harald N. Johnson, a staff member of the Rockefeller Foundation, observes, "On the basis of clinical evidence, there seems to be no doubt that rabies vaccine is effective in preventing the disease in the majority of the instances in which there is an expected incubation period of more than one month." But such an incubation period can only be expected in cases involving bites on the arms, legs, or torso. The chances that the Pasteur treatment will prevent the development of the disease when the victim is bitten severely on the head or neck are slight.

Only one more or less controlled test of rabies immunization in human beings has ever been made. That was conducted by a World Health Organization team in 1954, in Iran. Its purpose was to evaluate an antirabies serum developed that year by Hilary Koprowski, assistant director of viral and rickettsial research at the Lederle Laboratories of the American Cyanamid Company. Serum differs from vaccine in that it contains—rather than merely stimulates the body to produce—the immunizing agents known as antibodies. A rabid wolf had burst into a mountain village, not far from the W. H. O. team's station, and bitten twenty-nine men, women, and children. As a matter of course, the Pasteur treatment was prescribed at once for all the victims. In addition, seventeen of the group, whose wounds included bites on the head or neck, were given immediate injections of serum. Eleven of them received one injection, the others two or more. The results were unmistakably clear. Twenty-five of the victims, including all who had received at least two injections of serum, survived. Of the four who died, three had been given only the Pasteur treatment, and the other a single serum inoculation. The limited efficacy of the Pasteur treatment is not, unfortunately, its only flaw. It has others. It is unpleasantly long (the present regimen, even when supplemented by serum, requires from fourteen to twenty-one days), it is usually expensive (the average injection costs about five dollars), and, above all, it is disturbingly dangerous. Reactions to antirabies treatment range from those common in allergic conditions— erythematous or urticarial rashes, edema, syncope—to one known as neuroparalytic accident. Neuroparalytic accident varies in degree from a polyneuritis to ascending encephalomyelitis. The latter, in an uncomfortable number of cases, is permanently incapacitating, and sometimes fatal.

The imperfections of the Pasteur treatment are not, of course, sufficient to deny it a place in the modern medical kit. There is, after all, nothing with which to replace it. In the opinion of most investigators, however, the imperfections are pronounced enough to discourage its use in any but cases of certain—or suspicious but unverifiable —exposure. It is also their urgent conviction that post-exposure prophylaxis is, at best, an indirect defense against the menace of rabies. "There can be no question that the ultimate solution to the rabies problem is predicated on the control and eventual elimination of the disease from animal populations," the *American Journal of Public Health* commented editorially in May, 1955. "This may be accomplished by the setting up of transmission barriers, such as animal immunization, elimination of stray dogs, and the reduction of excessive numbers of wildlife vectors." It has been accomplished in a considerable number of countries. Britain, where a system of controls, rigidly enforced by the Ministry of Agriculture and Fisheries, was established around 1900, is perhaps the most notable of these. The last human exposure to rabies in England occurred nearly fifty years ago, and except for a handful of cases among imported dogs held in quarantine, there have been no outbreaks among animals there since shortly after the First World War. The Scandinavian countries—Denmark, Sweden, and Norway—have, by similar exertions, achieved almost as admirable a record, and so, among others, have Australia, New Zealand, and Malaya.

The record of the United States, despite the existence of an elaborate apparatus of legislative controls, is less imposing. Except for Hawaii, where rabies has somehow never gained a foothold, few parts of this country are wholly free of the disease. Last year, around half a million Americans were treated for bites inflicted by animals. Of these, sixty thousand were judged to have been exposed to rabies and received the Pasteur treatment. Three of them died. There were nine additional fatalities among persons who received incomplete or no treatment. The lowest incidence of human rabies in recent years was ten cases, in 1949. The highest was fifty-six cases, in 1944. Among domestic animals the average annual mortality is between seven and eight thousand. The persistence of rabies in man and beast throughout the United States has been variously explained, but two factors are considered decisive. One of these is indifference. Although many states have laws that specify a certificate of vaccination as a prerequisite for obtaining a dog license, and although all make some provision for the disposal of strays, such measures are seldom enforced, and then only in moments of epidemic panic. The other is the still enormous number of wild animals among which the rabies organism is endlessly perpetuated. This indigenous reservoir includes not only such conspicuous vectors as the fox and the skunk but badgers, raccoons, beavers, squirrels, and, since the early nineteen-fifties, the insectivorous bat.

The full significance of the bat attacks on Frances Roberts, Carl Dayton, David Bonner, and Mabel Tate has yet to be determined. One thing, however, seems certain.

These four people were not the victims of a fleeting freak of nature. Their experiences have since been duplicated elsewhere in the country. Three more attacks by rabid bats were reported in 1954. All occurred in Texas—the first, early in April, in San Antonio, and the second and third, in May and July, near Austin. The victims were a youth of twenty and two small children. Another was reported in October, 1955, in Madera, California, and involved a middle-aged man. Two more attacks—one certain and the other probable—were added to the record in 1956, and in May, 1957, an eleven-year-old boy was attacked near his home in Janesville, Wisconsin, and bitten on the arm and chin. The 1956 victims were a soldier on maneuvers in Louisiana and a Texas State Health Department field epidemiologist named George C. Menzies. Dr. Menzies, at the time of his exposure, had been collecting specimens of cave-dwelling bats in central Texas to be examined for evidence of rabies infection. How and when he was exposed is not known. It is only known that he returned to his home, in Austin, on January 1, and the following morning developed symptoms of rabies. Two days later he was dead. The six other victims received the Pasteur treatment, and survived.

Dr. Menzies's last assignment was one of a number of similar studies that have been undertaken in collaboration with the United States Public Health Service since the Bonner episode in 1953. The investigation, which was understandably intensified by the harrowing discovery at Carlsbad Caverns two years later, is expected to continue for at least another year. Some months will then be required to accurately assess its results. The preliminary findings, however, have been tentatively correlated by Ernest S. Tierkel, chief of Rabies Control Activities at the service's Communicable Disease Center, in Atlanta, and they are hardly reassuring. "During the last eighteen months or so, various field units have bagged in the neighborhood of ten thousand bats, in sixteen different states," Dr. Tierkel says. "About a hundred and fifty of them were positive for rabies. The group included four species of tree-living, or solitary, bats and eight species of cave-dwellers, or colonials. All, of course, insectivorous. Every state in which we've made a thorough study has yielded its quota of positives. The list, at the moment, is Alabama, California, Florida, Georgia, Louisiana, Michigan, Minnesota, Montana, New Mexico, New York, Ohio, Oklahoma, Pennsylvania, Texas, Utah, and Wisconsin. Those are the facts that we have to work with. What they mean—their epidemiological significance—is what we hope to find out.

"In the early phases of our investigation, one possible conjecture was that what we were turning up wasn't really rabies. We thought it might be a new virus disease of bats so closely related antigenically to the rabies virus that the two couldn't be differentiated by the usual laboratory tests. But a little more laboratory work disposed of that possibility. The disease is definitely rabies. Another basic question is whether the disease has always been present in the insectivorous bats of the United States and we have only just discovered it, or whether it represents a recent northward invasion into this country from the vampire-bat-rabies areas in Latin America. I'm inclined to suspect that the latter is the answer. We know, at any rate, that the Mexican free-tails of our Southwest migrate deep into the vampire country of Mexico. According to some authorities, the vampires and the free-tails even share the same winter caves. We hope that's all they share. If it turns out, as some preliminary findings have suggested, that our bats also share the vampires' resistance to rabies, we're up against an extremely difficult problem. Vampires—some of them, at least—are known to be capable of transmitting the disease for long periods of time without showing any signs of illness themselves. In other words, they're like Typhoid Mary. They're true carriers. If our bats have that capacity, if we find that they sometimes attack simply because they're frightened and not because they've been driven into a frenzy by the disease, and if we also find that the bat represents an important reservoir of rabies in the United States . . . Well, those are only possibilities, of course. We don't have the data yet to even hazard an answer. But what if they're shown to be facts? I think it would be a very good idea to tighten up our system of rabies controls."

One of the Lucky Ones

AMONG the more obviously ailing suppliants who appeared at Mount Sinai Hospital, on upper Fifth Avenue, on the afternoon of Tuesday, February 15, 1949, was a man I'll call Arnold Schneider. Schneider was only thirty-seven years old, but that day he could have passed for sixty-five or seventy. His back was bent, his gait was slow and shuffling, and his hands, his face, and the whites of his eyes were a ghastly lemon yellow. He felt as wretched as he looked. He had a blinding headache, he told the examining physician, there was a burning pain in the pit of his stomach, and he was dizzy, diarrheic, and nauseated—violently nauseated. He hadn't had a bite to eat since Sunday. The very thought of food was enough to double him up. To the best of his recollection, it was Sunday night, at supper, that his trouble had begun. Nothing had tasted right. Also, he had felt tired and his bones had ached. His wife suggested that he probably had a touch of the flu. He thought so, too. So, to be on the safe side, as soon as they had cleared the table and done the dishes he went straight to bed. A few hours later, around midnight, he had an attack of cramps, and vomited. That seemed to help, and Monday morning he felt a trifle better. Enough at least, to get up. But on the way to work—he owned a half interest in a cleaning and pressing shop on West Ninety-sixth Street, just down the street from his flat—he had another seizure, and it was all he could do to get back home. Since then, he had been in almost constant misery. What really worried him, though, was his urine. It was dark brown, almost black. He had never heard of such a thing. This morning was the first time he had noticed it, and it had sent him, as rapidly as he could drag himself into his clothes and around the corner, to the nearest doctor. The doctor had sent him to the hospital. Schneider reached in his pocket and brought out an envelope. Here was a note from the doctor. The examining physician smiled a reassuring smile, glanced at the note, and clipped it to an admittance form. Apart from identifying its author as a man of conventional prudence, the message told him nothing that he hadn't known since the patient entered the room. Schneider, as his color alone made pitifully plain, had jaundice.

The following morning, after a fitful night in an observation ward, Schneider was roused, raised, and rolled away for a barrage of diagnostic tests and soundings. That was routine but imperative. Jaundice is a morbid condition, and often a serious one, but it is not in itself a disease. Like chills and fever and malaise, it is merely a sign of disease. The immediate cause of jaundice is an excess of bile pigment in the blood. Since the manufacture, the storage, and the discharge of bile (a citreous fluid essential to the digestive process) are functions of some of the body's most highly specialized organs, a bilious complexion is rather more than disfiguring. It inevitably signals one or another of three largely distinct debilities. One of these is a derangement of the cells of the liver. A second is an obstruction in the bile duct. The third is a catastrophic destruction of red corpuscles. By the time Schneider was back in bed again it was clear to the resident in charge of the study that both a blocked duct and a blood breakdown could safely be eliminated as possible sources of trouble. That narrowed it down to the liver. A little past noon, the final returns came in from the laboratory, and they narrowed it down still further. Schneider's liver was ravaged in a manner that could have been accomplished only by some sudden, shattering assault. The resident took a brief turn among the now comfortably limited alternatives and uncapped his pen. He entered on the record a tentative diagnosis of acute infectious—or virus—hepatitis.

Some four or five hours later, on his evening tour of inspection, the attending physician was brought at first sight to much the same conclusion. The clinical findings, as enumerated on the chart in the ward nurse's office, were all in excellent harmony with a reading of hepatogenous jaundice. So, he soon satisfied himself, was the general appearance of the patient. Schneider lay as limp as a string—oblivious, apparently, to everything but pain. After a moment of silence and sympathy, the doctor turned away, toward the next of his scheduled stops. But halfway, he halted, arrested by a freak of perception. He then swung around and walked thoughtfully back up the ward to the office. Unless his memory was completely confused, there was an entry in the record that rendered it less than likely that Schneider's hepatitis stemmed from a virus infection. The record had been returned to the file, but he found it without any trouble and drew out the opening page. He hadn't been mistaken. The notation was there, just below the patient's name, age, and address. It read, "Occupation: dry cleaner." The doctor sat down at the desk and picked up the telephone and called the administration office. He asked the clerk who took his call to notify, the first thing in the morning, the Division of Industrial Hygiene and Safety Standards of the New York State Department of Labor—an agency, at 80 Centre Street, whose functions include the prompt and thorough investigation of any illness anywhere in the state that appears to be occupational in origin—that the hospital had under treatment a case of what looked very much like carbon-tetrachloride poisoning.

Some sixty million people in the United States, or a trifle over half the total adult population, are regularly employed in industry, business, agriculture, and the professions. Their presence on the job, however, is somewhat less than regular. Every day in the year, at least a million and a half of them are absent from work because of sickness. Of this number, a considerable minority—perhaps two hundred thousand—are victims of more than the common run of aches and pains and contagions that harry mankind. Their ailments are a natural, if not an unavoidable, result of the nature of their work. Occupational disease is a peculiarly sinister source of human misery. It is also an inexhaustible one. None of the astronomically various methods by which man makes his living is wholly without some hazard to physical or mental health. The fisherman's rheumatism, the waiter's fallen arches, the surgeon's hypertension, the miner's silicosis, the boilermaker's deafness, the bus driver's peptic ulcer, and the housemaid's bursitic knee are all, like a thousand other complaints, more or less directly attributable to the environmental conditions under which their victims work. The scope of occupational disease is vast almost beyond calculation. In one or another of its several entities, it sounds practically the full scale of physiologic, biochemic, and metabolic disharmonies known to modern medicine. It comes, in fact, unpleasantly close to being the major public-health problem of our time, and is probably the most permanent.

Like most diseases, those of occupational origin are distinguished not by their manifestations but by their causes. They differ, however, from those of general incidence in two important respects. One is that their causes all are pretty well known. The other is that they are all—potentially, at least—preventable. That they continue to occur with formidable frequency can be laid only partly to greed or need or carelessness. Nor is their awesome abundance and variety much of a factor. Their persistence is due largely to the fact that there are few such diseases whose presenting signs and symptoms unmistakably reflect their cause. In most, the clinical evidence can be anything but etiologically illuminating. It is often even misleading. For, in one way or another, most occupational diseases resemble with striking exactness one or another of the rather more familiar disorders. As a result, except among physicians trained in industrial medicine they are seldom recognized—and hence seldom reported and investigated—for what they are.

Despite its encyclopedic reach, most authorities recognize just four basic sources of occupational disease. Their roots, though occasionally entwined, are perceptibly distinct. One is emotional stress. Physical stress (heat, cold, damp, noise, glare, vibration, radiant energy) is, of course, another. A third is infection—anthrax, tularemia, undulant fever. Of these three fundamental hazards, only the first (inasmuch as it can spring with equal ease from fear, anxiety, or brain-washing boredom) is of compellingly wide significance, and together they probably account for little more than fifty per cent of all cases. The other source of occupational disease is poison. A poison may enter the body by way of the mouth, the lungs, or the skin. Its usual conduit in outbreaks among the general population is the gastrointestinal tract. In industrial poisoning, it follows a different itinerary. The mouth is seldom the portal of entry, and passage through the skin is only a trifle less rare. It almost always makes its entrance through the respiratory system.

There are literally thousands of substances whose dusts or vapors are toxic. They include most heavy metals, many coal-tar distillates and hydrocarbon derivatives, and certain natural or combustion gases. Some of them have menaced man for centuries. From the earliest hours of civilization, the asphyxiating powers, if not the nature, of such products of decomposing vegetable matter as carbon dioxide and hydrogen sulfide have been painfully familiar to miners, well diggers, and other burrowers underground. Both these gases are sluggish, inconspicuous, and tend to accumulate in pockets. Carbon dioxide, whose generation depletes the oxygen in the air, is known to mineworkers as black (or choke) damp, and their use of mice, canaries, or lighted candles to detect its presence is among the most venerable techniques of industrial-disease control. Hydrogen sulfide, in the popular vocabulary, is sewer gas. Unlike carbon dioxide, which has only a faint and scratchy odor, it emits a warning stench, (the rotten-egg smell common to all sulfur compounds), but this forthright characteristic is more than offset by its nearly instantaneous action. In Texas, in 1929, a whim of the wind drew a cloud of hydrogen sulfide from an oil well and blew it into a nearby herd of mules. The animals were dead before they could wheel and bolt.

Carbon monoxide has at least as long a history. It is formed by the incomplete combustion of some carbonaceous material (wood, coal, petroleum) and has been a hazard to man since the domestication of fire. It is violently toxic (ten times more so than carbon dioxide), it is uniquely versatile (no other gas is so capable of inducing both chronic and acute reactions), and it is by far the most insidious of all asphyxiants. For all practical purposes, carbon monoxide is indistinguishable from air. It has almost exactly the same free-flowing buoyancy, and it is equally colorless, odorless, and tasteless. Moreover, its inhalation, its passage through the lungs to the blood stream, and its accumulation there, where it displaces oxygen in the hemoglobin molecule, are seldom accompanied by any reliably alerting discomfort. Its action is less equivocal. An exposure of even five minutes to air containing as little as one per cent of carbon monoxide is almost always fatal. Chronic poisoning (marked by persistent headache, frequent vertigo, and sometimes, a progressive anemia) can result from prolonged daily exposure to concentrations of less than one fifth of one per cent. The gas is also ferociously plentiful. Its sources, though they have always been abundant, are now rapidly approaching the ubiquitous. Carbon monoxide is generously present in the effluvia of all internal-combustion engines, most industrial plants, and many mines, mills, and workshops. In automobile-exhaust fumes, for example, it averages about seven per cent. Because of the widespread installation of safety devices (fans, baffles, alarm meters), most cases of carbon-monoxide poisoning in industry these days are chronic, rather than acute, and even these are generally attributable to accidents. Industrial toxicologists are persuaded that thousands of workers—particularly automobile mechanics and storage-garage jockeys—suffer some degree of intoxication every day. Traffic policemen have lately been added to the list. A recent survey in Philadelphia demonstrated the presence of carbon monoxide in the blood of fourteen members of a downtown traffic squad. In six of these men, the amount ranged from twenty to thirty per cent. Anything much over ten per cent is usually considered dangerous.

Metal poisoning is almost entirely an occupational phenomenon. Except for an occasional freakish accident, its appearances outside industry are invariably either homicidal or suicidal in origin. They are just as invariably sudden and shattering, and, unless the poison, which always enters the body through the mouth, is eliminated by immediate vomiting, invariably end in death. In industry, metal poisoning is rarely, if ever, fatal. This is not, however, much cause for jubilation since, on the other hand, it is chronic, systemic, and, sometimes, incurable. Among the many metals whose fumes (or dusts) can seldom be inhaled with impunity, lead and mercury are notorious. White phosphorus (which, though not a metal, toxicologists find it convenient to classify as one) has much the same reputation. It shares with lead and mercury an inimitable capacity for highly specialized destruction. Phosphorus has a predilection for the jawbones, the gums, and the teeth. Long exposure to its fumes produces a necrotic condition known as "phossy jaw." This is characterized by a grotesque enlargement of the lower face and a slow, agonizing dissolution of the teeth. In severe cases, its spread throughout the body often can be checked only by the surgical removal of the entire jaw. Phossy jaw was once a common consequence of steady employment in a match factory. Since shortly before the First World War, when the manufacture of white-phosphorus matches was universally prohibited, its victims have been largely confined to workers in chemical, fertilizer, and ore-reduction plants.

Mercury has the distinction of inspiring the first attempt on record to control occupational disease by legislation. That was the passage of a law limiting the work of men employed in mercury mines at Idrija, in what is now Yugoslavia, to a maximum of six hours a day. It became effective in April of 1665. Chronic mercury poisoning, or mercurialism, was well known long before that time, certainly since the first Christian century. (The writings of Plutarch contain a rebuke to a mineowner for using slaves in his mercury mines who were not also criminals.) It could hardly have failed to be. Like phosphorus poisoning, the damage it inflicts is only too apparent. Mercury strikes at the central nervous system. With one exception (a pyorrheal inflammation of the mouth), the dominant signs of mercurialism all have a neural cast. Two are sufficiently singular to require specific listing in most medical dictionaries. One of them is a progressive intention tremor called hatter's shakes. The other is a personality derangement for which an eighteenth-century English investigator coined the term "erethism." Erethism is marked by constant anxiety, black depression, and alternating spells of infantile timidity and savage irritability. Sometimes, in advanced cases, its victims are racked by nightmare hallucinations, and even near-epileptic convulsions have been reported. The tremor of mercurialism takes its name from the trade that has always been a major source of the disease. Until about a generation ago, when several less toxic substitutes were devised, mercury was an essential ingredient in the processing of felt for hats. The use of mercury in hatmaking is now illegal in many European countries and in most American states. In less enlightened parts of the world, about the only defense available to hatters is chewing tobacco. Many hatters believe, though without much justification, that constant spitting will eliminate the poisonous fumes. Hatter's shakes first affects the muscles of the eyelids, the fingers, and the tongue. It then moves on to the arms and legs. In time, its victims may become wholly incapacitated—unable to eat, dress, or walk without assistance. The saying "mad as a hatter" and the Mad Hatter of *Alice in Wonderland* both derive from the lurching gait, the tangled tongue, and the addled wits of mercurialism.

Lead poisoning, or plumbism (the terms derives from *plumbum*, the Latin word for "lead"), has also enriched our literature, though rather less conspicuously. Its clinical manifestations are celebrated in *Alexipharmaca*, one of the two surviving works of the pre-Christian Greek poet Nicander. The poem reads, in part:

> The mouth it [lead] inflames and makes cold from
>   within,
> The gums dry and wrinkled are parch'd like the skin,
> The rough tongue feels harsher, the neck muscles
>   grip,
> He soon cannot swallow, foam runs from his lip,
> A feeble cough tries it in vain to expel,
> He belches so much, and his belly does swell. . . .

Meanwhile there comes a stuporous chill,
His feeble limbs droop and all motion is still.

As Nicander intimated, and numerous cooler clinicians
have subsequently confirmed, muscular atrophy, abdomi-
nal distention, and a curious stippling of the gums are
classically suggestive of plumbism. The first of these (it
usually takes the form of a limp, or "dropped," wrist)
and the last (a dark-blue line, somewhat resembling a
tattoo) always point to the presence of lead in the body.
They are not, however, always, or even often, present.
The usual seat of plumbism is the gastrointestinal laby-
rinth, and its usual indications are bloat and prolonged
paroxysms of almost unendurable pain. The deranging
colic can be subdued by prompt medication, but since
it stems from a massive accumulation of lead in the body,
usually absorbed (as dust or fumes) over a long period
of time, such treatment is essentially only palliative. Unless the lead can be dissolved (by means of a most complex procedure) and excreted, the gassy pains tend to
recur. The gum discoloration is permanent. So, if firmly
established, is the characteristic palsy. During the past
twenty-five years, largely as a result of educating workers, the incidence of plumbism has perceptibly declined,
but the disease is still far from conquered. It still seizes
hundreds, if not thousands, of victims every year. Its persistence, though hardly inevitable, is understandable
enough. No metal is more widely used than lead. It is
encountered in most of the traditional trades (painting,
printing, plumbing, mining, pottery making) and in
many of recent origin. Altogether, according to the
United States Department of Labor, some exposure to
lead occurs in a hundred and fifty different occupations.

The exact number of occupations that involve the use
of one or another of the coal-tar distillates and hydrocarbon derivatives is not known. New ones turn up too
fast for ready computation. The only certainty is that

these cabalistically complicated substances dominate modern industry. At least two hundred of them are now in general use. The most broadly serviceable compounds include benzol (or coal-tar benzene), beta-naphthylamine, carbon disulfide, carbon tetrachloride, and dinitrophenol. Most of this group figure importantly in the manufacture of numerous essentials of twentieth-century culture (mechanical refrigerators, lubricating oils, rubber cement, aniline dyes, plastics, explosives, and artificial silk), and all are incomparable solvents. They possess to perfecton all the qualities that make a dry cleaner efficient. Their cost is low, their volatility (or speed of evaporation) is high, and their avidity for fats and greases is insatiable. They are also, however, almost incomparably toxic. The fumes of carbon disulfide derange the nervous system. Exposure to benzol vapor may produce the lethally wasting condition known as aplastic anemia. A possible result of beta-naphthylamine poisoning is cancer of the bladder. Dinitrophenol, which was once the effective essense of a popular reducing drug, has the power to race the metabolism to the point of irreparable collapse. Carbon tetrachloride is less narrowly selective. The areas to which it is drawn include the heart, the bowels, the lungs, the kidneys, and the liver.

The kaleidoscopic range of carbon tetrachloride is not its only distinction. It has, unfortunately, others. It is particularly partial to the overfed, the undernourished, and the alcoholic (the presence of even a small amount of alcohol in the blood will enormously intensify its action), and, with the possible exception of benzol, it is the most reliably ravaging of all familiar solvents. It is in addition, as the attending physician at Mount Sinai Hospital was nicely aware that February evening in 1949, the one most highly esteemed by a majority of American dry cleaners. The reason for its popularity is anything but arbitrary. It could hardly be more practical. Unlike benzol, beta-naphthylamine, carbon disulfide, and dinitrophenol, all of which will burst into flame at a spark, carbon tetrachloride is as incombustible as soapy water.

The report on Arnold Schneider was telephoned to the Division of Industrial Hygiene and Safety Standards of the New York State Department of Labor on Thursday morning, February 17. As is customary, it was received and promptly recorded there by a clerk in the Medical Unit. That was around eight o'clock. When a physician on the staff of the unit—whose name, at his request, shall here be Paul Temple—reached the office some twenty minutes later, a memorandum containing the facts of the case (the name, address, and occupation of the patient, and the nature of his trouble and its suspected source) was lying on his desk. He read it with interest, and a kind of satisfaction.

"I don't mean to sound inhuman," Dr. Temple says. "Actually, my reaction was quite the reverse of heartless. I was simply gratified, as we always are down here, to learn that somebody in general medicine was thinking in terms of occupational disease. Most doctors in ordinary practice don't. That's only natural, of course. It's outside their field of training and experience. The possibility that the kind of work the patient does may be a vital factor in the problem just doesn't occur to them. Not very often, anyway. They tend to concentrate entirely on the clinical picture. That can be very misleading. It can even be fatal. The industrial diseases are pretty tricky. And not only because their symptoms are rarely pathognomonic. A clinically accurate diagnosis isn't enough. Neither is the best of treatment. Unless the fundamental cause is known, it's little better than nothing. It hardly suffices to save a man's life and then, because it never dawned on anybody to relate his job to his illness, let him go right back to the environment that sent him to the hospital in the first place. That isn't very successful therapeutics. It isn't very good preventive medicine either.

"But in this case, apparently, the truth had dawned. Somebody had made a differential diagnosis on the basis of all the available facts. That was most refreshing. So I was pleased, and relieved. Not, of course, that I accepted the diagnosis as fact. Carbon-tetrachloride poisoning was merely the most reasonable assumption. In still had to be proved. But one thing, at least, was certain. Arnold Schneider was one of the lucky ones. From our standpoint, anyway. When and if he recovered, it would be permanent. He wouldn't come tottering back to the hospital in a couple of weeks with the same thing all over again. No matter what the cause of his trouble turned out to be. An attack of infectious hepatitis confers a fairly lasting immunity, and physical agents can be controlled. He would be safe. Moreover, and no less importantly, if the hospital was right, so would everyone else who worked in his cleaning establishment. We could see to that. And at once. Prevention is our first concern. Well, in this case that presented no problem. We knew where to begin. We had the suspected source. A look around the shop should answer a good many questions. That phase of our work is handled by the Chemical Unit. I called William J. Burke, the chief of the unit, and gave him the information I had. The rest was a matter of routine. One of his men would take it from there. I'd have the results as soon as he made his report.

"For the moment, that was that. There was nothing to do right now but wait. Our next move would depend on what we found at the shop. An investigation of the kind that was indicated here takes time. I didn't expect to hear from Burke for several hours, and I didn't. It was almost two when he called. He sounded puzzled. I must say he had his reasons. The findings at the shop were hardly what I'd led him to expect. Quite the contrary. The chemist assigned to the job had camped in the shop all morning. He had watched the work and examined the apparatus and made every possible test, and ended up in a glow. His report was practically a testimonial. Schneider and his partner—Thompson was his name—were one among many. Their shop was everything most dry-cleaning shops aren't. It was a model. The equipment was the best and the safest on the market. It was a single-vat machine, airtight and fully automatic. All the operator himself did was put in the clothes and take them out. Everything else—the introduction of the solvent, the cleaning and drying operations, and the extraction and disposal of the solvent—was controlled by buttons and levers. Also, the machine was almost new. They had been in business only a little over a year. There was just one point at all in line with expectations. The solvent they used was carbon tetrachloride. Under the circumstances, however, that didn't really signify. The chemist had run a test on the air in the shop. It showed a ratio of something like twenty parts of carbon tet to a million parts of air. The accepted maximum in New York State is thirty-five. In some states, anything under a hundred is considered safe enough. Well, that took care of that. I thanked Burke and hung up. The shop was out.

"I can't truthfully say I was sorry. As an industrial hygienist, I was bound to feel encouraged. A good shop is always good news. Still, I wasn't exactly elated. It didn't go very far toward explaining Schneider's trouble. Unless, of course, I took it to mean that his illness and his occupation were totally unrelated. In that event, as far as we were concerned, the case was closed. But I couldn't. I simply wasn't willing to dismiss the fact that he worked in a place where carbon tetrachloride was used as merely an odd coincidence. Not yet, at any rate. Besides, there was that diagnostician at Mount Sinai. He had made a very sensible deduction. It would be nice to justify his alertness. And then I was curious. I just plain wanted to know. But the trouble was there was nothing I myself could do about it. I was involved in a couple of other things that would keep me in the office all afternoon. I checked the schedule, and one of the other medical investigators was free. He's in private practice now, so I'll say his name was Boone. I called him in and he was interested, and we talked it over. That didn't take us long. There was only one real question. If Schneider did have toxic hepatitis—if it really was a case of carbon-tetrachloride poisoning—how and where was he exposed? Or, rather, if the shop was eliminated, where did we start? Boone didn't agree that the shop was definitely out. He wanted to see for himself. A talk with Thompson might put him on to something that a chemist could very easily overlook.

"But the shop *was* out. Thompson settled that. Boone called back in about an hour and gave me the story. It couldn't have been more conclusive. It would have finished the shop as a possible source even without the chemical report. Schneider had nothing to do with the mechanical end of the business. That was Thompson's department. Schneider worked up front. He kept the books and made deliveries and waited on the trade. So if there had been some kind of accident in the workroom—I gathered that's what Boone had had in mind—our victim wouldn't be Schneider. It would be Thompson. But Thompson was the picture of health. And there hadn't been any accident.

"Boone was still at the shop when he phoned. His next stop, of course, was the hospital. Schneider himself seemed the only lead we had left. If, that is, he was still alive and could talk. Well, it turned out that he was and could, and did. Just barely—although he had managed to round the corner and was off the critical list—but enough. However, I didn't know that for some little time—not until almost six o'clock. I'd finally cleared my desk and was ready to call it a day when the phone rang. It was Boone. It was all over. He had it all tied up. The tone of his voice told me that. I sat down and waited for him to tell me the rest. He was calling from the Schneider apartment. Mrs. Schneider, whom he had met at the hospital, was with him. So was the source. I saw it the next day, on a shelf in the chemical lab. It was a gallon jug about two thirds full of carbon tetrachloride. Schneider had filled it from a drum at the shop on Saturday and brought it home that night. The living-room rug needed cleaning. On Sunday afternoon, around three o'clock, he emptied part of the jug into a pail, dug up a scrubbing brush, and went to work. It was a wall-to-wall carpet, and what with shifting the furniture around and stopping every now and then to rest, the job took a couple of hours. I must say Boone gave me the picture. An open pail of carbon tet, a dripping brush, and Schneider down on his hands and knees with his face about a foot from the rug—it made my hair stand on end. It also made me wonder. It settled the question of Schneider, all right. But it raised another question.

" 'What about Mrs. Schneider?' I asked.

" 'Oh,' Boone said. 'She's fine. She wasn't at home that afternoon. She was up in the Bronx, or somewhere, visiting her mother. But it probably wouldn't have mattered either way. It's a good-sized room, with doors opening into the rest of the flat. Also, Schneider knew enough to open a couple of windows. What he didn't know was something else. While he was working, he had a bottle of beer, maybe two. He isn't sure which.'

" 'One could be plenty,' I said.

" 'Yes,' said Boone. 'And when he began to feel rotten and got into bed, his wife fixed him a nice hot toddy.' "

$CH_3CO_2C_6H_4CO_2H$

AROUND five o'clock on the afternoon of Wednesday, May 4, 1955, an office boy walked into the office of Dr. Harold Jacobziner, Assistant Commissioner for Maternal and Child Health of the New York City Health Department and chief of the department's newly established Poison Control Center, with a memorandum initialed by a clerk in the report room of the center. Dr. Jacobziner had his hat on his head and his briefcase in his hand, but the message turned him back to his desk. He sat down, glanced again at the paper, and paused for a moment of geographical calculation. Then he picked up the telephone and dialed the department's Bureau of Public Health Nursing. An official of his acquaintance answered the call, and after a brisk exchange of civilities Dr. Jacobziner got briskly down to business. He had a job for one of the nurses on the staff of the municipal health center that served the Corona section of Queens. The assignment was an investigatory visit to the home of a couple named (I'll say) Mr. and Mrs. Francis R. Poole. They lived at —Alburtis Avenue, in Corona. According to a formal notification just received by the Poison Control Center, their son, a boy of three named Richard, had been admitted to Whitestone Memorial Hospital a few hours earlier. It was another case of acute acetylsalicylic-acid intoxication.

Acetylsalicylic acid is the universal comforter known in the Esperanto of the laboratory as $CH_3CO_2C_6H_4CO_2H$ and almost everywhere else as aspirin. The latter is a term of proprietary origin that has achieved an all but total nomenclatural ascendancy over science. This triumph, though unique in medical history, was in no way uniquely accomplished. In common with all such fabrications that have outgrown the stigma of trade, the widespread acceptance of the name is generally attributable to its distinctive sound, to its attractive brevity, and to many years of pertinacious advertising. Nevertheless, unlike much commercial coinage, "aspirin" is not altogether an etymological freak. Its lineage is acceptably legitimate. It derives, roughly but rationally, from *Spiraea*, a botanical genus whose more prominent members (bridal wreath, meadow-sweet, hardhack) are natural sources of salicylic acid, the active principle in aspirin. As it happens, however, the vegetable secretion of the acid is far from confined to plants of the *Spiraea* group. It also occurs in many other shrubs (jasmine, madder, patridgeberry), and in many legumes (peas, beans, clover), grasses (wheat, rye, sugar cane), and trees (beech, birch, olive, poplar, willow). The *Spiraea* were merely among the first such plants to be identified by modern pharmacology.

That the bark, fruit, and leaves of these plants contain some revitalizing agent has long been common, if largely rustic, knowledge. Potions rich in salicylic acid are as old as herbal therapy, and almost as ubiquitous. Practically all races seem to have early grasped their usefulness. A draught whose ingredients included the juice of willow bark was esteemed by many North American Indian tribes as an antipyretic, or fever reducer. Another aboriginal people—the Hottentots of South Africa—made good use of an essentially similar decoction to ease the agony of rheumatism. The willow, among other salicylate plants, was also held in high regard throughout the early

Mediterranean world. Hippocrates, in the fourth century before Christ, recognized its capacity for relieving both pain and fever. He also perspicaciously recommended topical applications of willow leaves, presumably as an antiseptic, in the *post-partum* care of maternity cases, and, less perspicaciously, the juice of poplar bark for various eye diseases. A generation later, Theophrastus, a pioneer botanist who succeeded Aristotle as head of the Lyceum at Athens, proclaimed the analgesic excellence of madder bark. He was, in addition, commendably inspired to urge the inclusion of madder in the manual of mild but effective diuretics. Theophrastus's success in thus broadening the therapeutic range of the salicylates was presently matched by other investigators. Around A.D. 75, Dioscorides, a Greek surgeon in Roman military service, rose from a series of experiments with the discovery that a paste composed of willow ash would safely remove such callosites as corns. In the course of this study, he had stumbled upon the further fact that his corn cure was almost as useful in combating the torments of gout. Pliny the Elder, the celebrated Roman encyclopedist, placed willow juice on the diuretic list. He then went on to propose an infusion of poplar bark as a specific for sciatica, and, amending, if not improving upon, Hippocrates, suggested poplar gum to druggists in search of a satisfactory eyewash. To these innovations, more imaginative minds rapidly added an unguent of willow bark as a cure for earache, one of willow leaves as a dressing for bloody wounds, and a willow poultice to dissipate fistulas and erysipelatous lesions. By the end of the second century, when Galen completed his valiant thirty-volume pharmacopoeia, all the remedial powers—great, small, illusory— of the salicylates had been noted and defined. Galen was the mightiest of the Greco-Roman empirical pharmacists. He was also the last pharmacist of any stature anywhere until almost modern times. With the foundering of Rome, the whole of rational herbal therapy was lost to most of the Western world in the mists of Christian mysticism for well over a thousand years. "All diseases of Christians are to be ascribed to demons," St. Augustine announced in the fifth century.) But for a scattering of practical folkphysicians, too simple to comprehend the complexities of fashionable piety, it might well have been lost forever.

The classic grasp of botanical medicine managed to survive both Imperial Rome and the Holy Roman Empire only in the country kitchen. Among salicylate plants, the willow was the first to be recalled to the attention of science. An eighteenth-century English clergyman and naturalist named Edward Stone is usually considered its rediscoverer. His find, though unexpected, was not entirely adventitious. He knew, in a way, just what he was looking for. Stone, like many others of his time and inquisitive bent, had long diverted himself with the hope of finding in some common plant an inexpensive antipyretic substitute for Peruvian bark (or cinchona), as quinine was then called. One afternoon in 1763, while enjoying a rural ramble, he got wind of the fact (possibly during a pause in a country kitchen) that willow bark was locally much admired as a household remedy for the feverish chills of ague. A hint was all he needed. He sampled a piece of bark, found that it shared with cinchona an "extraordinary bitterness," and buckled down to work. Some months later, in a letter to the president of the Royal Society of London for Improving Natural Knowledge, he summarized his findings. His paper began with a word on the willow. "As this tree," he noted, "delights in a moist or wet soil, where agues chiefly abound, the general maxim, that many natural maladies carry their cures along with them, or that their remedies lie not far from their causes, was so very apposite to this particular case, that I could not help applying it; and that this might be the intention of Providence here, I must own, had some little weight with me." Then, having delivered himself of this rather shaky ratiocination, Stone got firmly down to cases. Providence had provided him with fifty of them. All were victims of "agues, and intermitting disorders," and although their seizures varied in severity, all were placed on the same regimen—twenty grains of powdered willow bark dissolved in a dram of water, administered every four hours. The results, he was happy to record, had been uniformly excellent.

Stone's triumphant report, which was presently published in the *Philosophical Transactions* of the Royal Society, had two triumphant results. The first, and by far the more direct and immediate, was a burst of corroborative clinical tests that promptly returned the willow to a reputable place in the professional medicine chest. The other was the introduction of the willow into the laboratories of scientific chemistry, which were then just opening. There, in the first decades of the nineteenth century, it happened to catch the eye of a cosmopolitan company of investigators whose particular interest was the chemical composition of medically useful plants. Their attention, once focused, was almost at once productive. The effective essence of willow bark was identified by the Italian chemists Fontana and Brugnatelli in 1826. Three years later, a French experimental pharmacist, Henri Leroux, accomplished its isolation. In 1838, the extraction of salicylic acid was accomplished by the Italian chemist Rafelle Piria. At about the same time, in Switzerland, an apothecary named Pagenstecher found that it could also be obtained from meadowsweet and bridal wreath, and his provocative find was closely followed by a succession of explorations, in England, Germany, and elsewhere, that quickly established its presence in a multitude of other plants. The inquiry then came to a halt. For it was almost as quickly established that salicylic acid, despite its abundance of sources, was too costly to extract to be of much practical use. Also, for the moment, the investigators had satisfied their curiosity.

Their curiosity remained quiescent for close to a generation. It revived, like the whole of organic chemistry, with the stentorian enunciation, by the German chemists Friedrich Wöhler and Justus von Liebig, of the theory of synthesis, or the interrelation of organic and inorganic substances. Among those who heard their call was a professor of chemistry at the University of Leipzig named Hermann Kolbe. To Kolbe, the sound was a summons. It summoned him to work, and to fame. In 1874, after a period of patient stalking, he emerged from his laboratory and held up to view in the pages of the *Journal für praktische Chemie* an economical procedure for the production of synthetic salicylic acid. The importance of Kolbe's achievement, which posterity has recorded as a milestone in the history of synthetics, was readily grasped by all but the most myopic, and the halls of progressive chemistry rang with appreciative applause. So, understandably, did those of contemporary medicine, but only for a time. The hopes it excited in medical science soon and suddenly withered. Although Kolbe had solved one practical problem, his solution brought another to light, which revealed itself at the first round of clinical trials. Pure salicylic acid, though a model of strength in dulling pain and banishing fever, was by no means a model drug. Its salubrious powers were more than offset by its high degree of toxicity. Large or frequent doses, the reporting clinicians agreed, almost always resulted in nausea, often in spasms of vomiting, and sometimes even in coma. The inquiry once more shifted its course. What was needed now, its participants perceived, was a neutralizing agent, or buffer. That meant searching out some substance that would combine with salicylic acid (not all elements are physiologically compatible), render it sufficiently bland for general clinical use, and yet leave unimpaired its therapeutic vigor. The chemists' resilience, for once, was fully and finally rewarded. There are, to the best of scientific knowledge, just three compounds that meet these requirements with anything approaching precision, and all were known and in service before the end of the century. One of them—sodium salicylate—turned up at the very first cast, in 1876. In 1885, the Polish pharmacologist Marcellus von Nencki identified phenyl salicylate as another. The third is acetylsalicylic acid. It was introduced in 1899.

Acetylsalicylic acid had its pharmacological origin in the laboratories of Friedrich Bayer & Company, later a subsidiary of I. G. Farbenindustrie, near Düsseldorf. It was first developed there, early in 1899, by a young research chemist named Felix Hoffmann. Hoffmann was not, nor did he claim to be, the actual discoverer of acetylsalicylic acid. That distinction had been achieved some forty years before by an Alsatian chemist named Charles Frédéric von Gerhardt. What Hoffmann discovered was its usefulness. Von Gerhardt had encountered acetylsalicylic acid in 1853 while exploring the interaction of various salts and acids, but he considered it merely a novelty. Like Paul Gelmo, the precocious Viennese student who in 1908 casually created and indifferently abandoned the coal-tar derivative known since its re-creation (by Gerhard Domagk, in 1933) as sulfanilamide, von Gerhardt was born too soon to comprehend what he had wrought. Hoffmann, like Domagk, was more favorably placed. His accomplishment, however, can be laid only partly to the instructive passage of time. He had other, less common advantages. Of these, two were decisive. One was a uniquely compelling source of inspiration in the person of his father. The elder Hoffmann was an invalid, a racked and crippled victim of rheumatoid arthritis. Of the remedies then at hand, including both sodium and phenyl salicylate, none could give him any adequate relief, and his life and become an agony. This wrenched the son from his workaday studies and drove him in search of some effective medicament. Hoffmann's other great gift was good luck. This guided his steps past the standard works in the scientific library to a compendium of chemical freaks and drones, and enabled him to find what he was looking for. His next move was conventional. Having satisfied himself, by laboratory test and domestic trial, of the worth of acetylsalicylic acid, he assembled his notes and carried them dutifully to the Bayer Company's director of pharmacological research. That was Heinrich Dreser, the architect of, among other things, diacetylmorphine, or heroin, and then an imposing figure in European science. Dreser reacted to the data set before him in a manner befitting his rank. He took one look, and took over. It was he who piloted acetylsalicylic acid through its first full-dress clinical evaluation. It was he who discarded its natural name as being hard to pronounce, hard to remember, and impossible to patent, and replaced it with the commercially seemlier "Aspirin." And it was he who wrote, and cheerfully signed, the pioneering report, confidently entitled "Pharmakologisches über Aspirin (Acetylsalicylsäure)," whose publication in *Pflügers Archiv für die gesamte Physiologie des Menschen und der Tiere* first brought the compound to the attention of medicine. That was toward the end of 1899. Its merits took it from there.

Acetylsalicylic acid (as most clinicians still choose to call it), or aspirin (the name practically everyone else prefers), or Aspirin (as its original proprietors were profitably privileged to insist on its being called until the general expiration of their patents around 1917), is an extraordinary drug. Almost everything about it is unusual. It comes, for one thing, impressively close to being the oldest therapeutic agent in continuing active demand. Only such venerable specifics as quinine (for malaria), colchicum (for gout), digitalis (for cardiac weakness), and, perhaps, the bromides (for relief of nervous tension) are of greater age and durability. Unlike these tottering centenarians, however, it has more than merely held its own against the massive ingenuities of mid-twentieth-century pharmacology. In 1935, the annual consumption of acetylsalicylic acid in the United States was estimated at four million pounds. By 1944, it had risen to nearly eight million. According to the least galvanic estimates, it now exceeds eleven million pounds, or, in terms of the standard dosage, approximately sixteen billion five-grain tablets. The true figure is probably well in excess of that, for, in general, such estimates refer only to the acetylsalicylic acid that is marketed under the name of aspirin. They seldom include that contained in the several more recently developed proprietary preparations—Bufferin, Anacin, Empirin, and Alka-Seltzer, among others—of which it is a major ingredient. The popularity of acetylsalicylic acid is almost equally immoderate elsewhere in the world. In some countries, notably Canada and those of Western Europe, it has, if anything, inspired an even fiercer veneration (England, for example, with hardly a fourth the population of the United States, consumes at least three million pounds of it a year), and there are no countries in which it is unknown, unappreciated, or unavailable. It is, in fact, the most widely used drug on earth. It is also the cheapest (a five-grain tablet costs about half a cent), one of the safest (many aspirant suicides have survived doses of more than two hundred grains), and, among drugs of a comparable nature, including its companion salicylates, without much doubt the best. Some authorities go further than that. They consider it the most generally useful drug in the entire armamentarium of medicine.

It is not hard to understand why. The great majority of drugs, as the heft of the modern pharmacopoeia is enough to suggest, are more conspicuous for the refinement than for the variety of their therapeutic feats. Hundreds, like insulin (the specific for *diabetes mellitus*) and heparin (an anticoagulant), are limited in usefulness to one particular function, and there are many hundreds

more whose present scope is only a trifle less narrow.
Even the widest-ranging antibiotics, for all the mul-
tiplicity of horrors—anthrax, brucellosis, endocarditis,
meningitis, tularemia, and syphilis, among others—over
which they have an almost sovereign domination, are anything but widely effective. Their range is wholly confined to diseases of infectious, or microbial, origin.
Acetylsalicylic acid is differently endowed. Although it
is incapable of mastering any disease, it possesses a master-
ful sweep. Few drugs embody more, or more various,
powers. As an analgesic, an antipyretic, an antirheumatic,
and—or at least so a recent study at the Boston University
School of Medicine, in which it appeared to show a
marked capacity for preventing the recurrence of kidney
stones, would suggest—an anticalculus, its palliative reach
embraces practically all the smaller miseries, as well as
some of those of considerable stature, that try the human
race.

Just how acetylsalicylic acid performs this symphony
of services has yet to be fully fathomed. Fifty years of investigation have illuminated little more than the general
route it follows through the body. Salicylic acid, the active principle of the drug, is absorbed directly from the
small intestine into the blood stream. It remains there,
moving with the current of the circulation, for, in most
cases, ten to fourteen hours. It then passes into the kidneys and is excreted in the urine. It is also known to
form in the kidneys a compound called glucuronide,
whose presence increases the solubility of calcium—a
phenomenon that would seem to explain its apparent an-
ticalculous action. The essential physiology of the acid
is otherwise very largely opaque. About the only further
probability is that each of its distinctive effects is achieved
by a different mechanism. There is no possible functional
connection between its capacity for generating glucuronide and any of its other attributes, and it seems almost
as certain that the processes by which it blocks pain, re-

duces fever, and suppresses joint inflammations are also completely unrelated. Of these three established powers, the first is the least mysterious. Most physiologists believe that the site of salicylic acid's analgesic action is the thalamus, the chief sensory reception center, located in the forebrain. There, in some obscure manner, the acid (or impulses set in motion by it) impedes the normal transmission of stimuli conveying the sensation of pain. The best evidence suggests that acetylsalicylic acid has the power to raise the threshold against pain perception by about thirty-five per cent. "A very small dose of aspirin has a measurable effect in raising the pain threshold," Stewart Wolf, head of the Department of Medicine of the University of Oklahoma School of Medicine, and Harold G. Wolff, professor of medicine at the Cornell University Medical College, noted in a recent monograph. "Increasing the dose has a progressively greater effect up to about ten grains, beyond which no additional pain-killing effect is manifest, although larger doses do somewhat prolong the duration of effect. With ten grains of aspirin, maximum effect is achieved in about one and a half hours. Thereafter its action in raising the pain threshold begins to dwindle. The effect can be kept at a peak most satisfactorily not by giving larger doses but by frequently repeating the ten-grain dose, say at two-hour intervals. . . . Combinations of analgesic drugs are no more effective than is the single strongest drug in the combination. The most that can be achieved in terms of deadening pain is the effect of ten grains of aspirin." This, of course, is not to say that acetylsalicylic acid is the strongest of all analgesics. It is merely the strongest that can be safely used without medical supervision. Morphine, for example, is capable of raising the threshold against pain perception as high as seventy per cent, but it also affects pain reaction; that is, it simultaneously blocks the passage of stimuli conveying such sensations as tension and anxiety. The artificial avoidance of tension and anxiety, is the basis of addition. Acetylsalicylic acid has no effect whatever on pain reaction.

Almost nothing is known about the way acetylsalicylic acid functions as a febrifuge. There are no absolute data on the dynamics involved, and only a few reasonably firm hypotheses. The firmest of these concern the general procedure by which a reduction of fever is accomplished. It was once held that the phenomenon could be ascribed largely to a braking action on the machinery of heat production. Recent research has substantially altered this view. The explanation now in vogue suggests that antipyresis results primarily from a simple quickening of the body's natural facilities for releasing excessive heat—the peripheral blood vessels and the sweat glands. Its ultimate cause, as currently envisioned, is more complex. Animal experiments have demonstrated that, contrary to snap assumption, this hyperactivity is induced not by direct stimulation of the superficial thermostatic apparatus but indirectly, through the central nervous system. In the opinion of most investigators, the specific focus of impact is probably one or another of the numerous regulatory nuclei that are clustered near the midbrain. Beyond this point, however, all suppositions falter. The nature of the power that acetylsalicylic acid has over these nuclei eludes even the nimblest imaginations, except for one twilit hypothesis: The control it exerts would seem to be somewhat less than total. For, as a mountain of empirical evidence makes clear, its influence is limited to remission of fever. It is peculiarly, and providentially, incapable, even in massive doses, of forcing the tempeturate of the body below 98.6 degrees, or normal.

Everything about the antirheumatic powers of acetylsalicylic acid is elusive. No one has any understanding of their fundamental character. It can be said only that they very definitely exist. They are, in fact, so plainly pronounced that acetylsalicylic acid has stood unchallenged for almost half a century as the drug of majority choice in the symptomatic treatment of rheumatic fever, rheumatoid arthritis, and other inflammations of connective tissue. Its position, though violently shaken by the cyclonic appearance of cortisone and ACTH in 1949, is still far from insecure. Many clinicians—especially in Britain, where the adrenocortical hormones were welcomed with a rather less millennial euphoria than in their native America—have never ceased to prefer it. "Modern hormone therapy notwithstanding, salicylate, either as the sodium salt or as acetylsalicylic acid—remains the safest and most satisfactory drug in the routine treatment of rheumatism," Stanley Graham, professor of child health at the University of Glasgow, wrote in a recent report to the *British Medical Journal*. Much the same opinion has been expressed by William McK. Jefferies, assistant professor of medicine at the Western Reserve University School of Medicine, in the *New England Journal of Medicine*. "Although ACTH, cortisone, or hydrocortisone in adequate doses can at least temporarily control the symptoms of rheumatoid arthritis in practically every case," Dr. Jefferies observed, "the chronic nature of this disease and the hazards of prolonged maintenance of steroid therapy make it generally advisable to try other accepted methods of treatment, such as salicylates and physiotherapy, first." To these views, Sir Henry Cohen and his fellow members of the Joint Committee of the (British) Medical Research Council and Nuffield Foundation on Clinical Trials of Cortisone, ACTH, and Other Therapeutic Measures in Chronic Rheumatic Diseases, which recently completed a definitive two-year study, have added the opinion that "for practical purposes there has been remarkably little to choose between cortisone and aspirin in the management of [rheumatoid arthritis]." Except, of course, as the committee must have felt it unnecessary to point out, in terms of price (the average effective dose of cortisone costs almost a dollar) and prudence.

Although, because of its low toxicity, its inability to dull the pain-reaction sense, and its lack of any effect on normal body temperature, acetylsalicylic acid ranks high among the safest of chemotherapeutic agents, it is by no means entirely innocuous. It has its savage side. Like most substances, including many foods, it can produce a variety of allergic reactions—dizziness, ear ringing, nausea, vomiting, skin eruptions, asthmatic seizures, muscular spasms—in susceptible individuals. Some of these idiosyncratics are so exquisitely responsive that a single grain can have a shattering, or even a fatal, impact. Cases have been reported of people's being thrown into convulsions upon receiving a blood tranfusion from a donor whose gift contained a just perceptible trace of the salicylate radical. Its touch can also dishevel constitutions that are not congenitally vulnerable. The cruel acidity that seriously flaws most salicylates is not altogether neutralized in the acetylsalicylic compounds. Chemistry has merely blunted its bite. There are certain diseases—peptic ulcer, for example, and coronary thrombosis—in which the use of acetylsalicylic acid may precipitate such complications as acute dyspepsia, prolonged retching, and hemorrhage. A general debility, such as that brought on by many essentially trivial ailments, may also, in a manner not yet fully understood, magnify its pernicious powers. It is, in addition, corrosive enough to sometimes enfeeble the most robustly well. No one can long consume immoderate amounts of aspirin (fifty or more grains a day) without suffering some degree of intoxication, and even a tablet or two, if swallowed whole on an empty stomach, often will cause a twinge of sour, heartburning discomfort. For all their abundance, however, the reprehensibly rash are not particularly prominent among those whom acetylsalicylic acid most commonly shakes or sickens. Nor, since they are generally made wary by early experience or experienced counsel, are the sensitive or the unwell. Its usual victims—in this country, at least — are children. According to the United States Food and Drug Administration, thousands of cases of salicylate poisoning of sufficient seriousness to require the services of a physician occur in the United States every year. In 1952, for instance, the total, including a hundred and thirteen cases that ended in death, reached nearly seventeen thousand. Of that number, nearly three fourths, or more than thirteen thousand, were children—young children. Hundreds were mere infants, a year old or less, and none was more than five. Most of them, like the boy whose case was brought to the attention of Dr. Jacobziner that afternoon last May, were around three.

The investigation into the case of Richard Poole that Dr. Jacobziner had requested fell to a visiting nurse named Veronica Flynn. Miss Flynn received the assignment when she reported for duty at the Corona District Health Center on Thursday morning, May 5, and she set about discharging it without excitement, or delay. A chronicle of her findings, which she wrote and posted late that afternoon, reached Dr. Jacobziner the following day. It made, he found, sad but familiar reading.

"I had fifteen others almost exactly like it in my files," Dr. Jacobziner said the other day. "All children, all accidents, all totally inexcusable. Only the details were different. Fifteen cases may not sound like very many. It wouldn't be today, of course. But it was then. In May, 1955, my file on acetylsalicylic-acid intoxication didn't go back very far. It only went back a couple of months— to the middle of March, in fact. That was when we established our Poison Control Center, with Harry Raybin, an extremely competent chemist, as its technical director. There wasn't any file on aspirin or any other kind of poisoning until then. The accumulation of epidemiological data is merely one phase of our work at the center. The function of the center is primarily educational. That takes two forms. One is to provide doctors and hospitals in the city with a source of accurate emergency information when they come up against some unfamiliar kind of poison. There are hundreds of potentially toxic chemical substances in daily household use. Every now and then, some child takes it into his head to sample one of them. In many instances, the doctor who gets the case has only the most general notion of what to do. He may know what it was that the child ate. That usually isn't much of a mystery. It was Johnson's Cream Furniture Wax, say, or Noxon Metal Polish, or Shinola. But he doesn't know what's in it. He doesn't know its chemistry. Our people do. When we get a call for help, we have the answer ready, and also the antidote, if any. In return for that service, however, we require something of the doctors and hospitals. They must notify us promptly of every case of chemical poisoning that comes to their attention. That's essential to the other aspect of our educational function. It gives us a chance to study the particular how and why of such outbreaks, and, often enough, to do something to prevent their recurrence. Well, the Poole case gave us something to study, all right. Not because it was unusual in any of its particulars. In that respect, as I say, Miss Flynn's report was only too familiar. It didn't tell us much of anything that we didn't already know about the causes of acetylsalicylic-acid poisoning. What made it a study was this: There was almost nothing that is known about the problem that wasn't present. It was practically a model of carelessness, bad luck, and ignorance.

"Miss Flynn's report was also something of a model. It couldn't have been more explicit. She began with a note on the boy. He was still at Whitestone Memorial, and his condition, at the moment of writing, was listed as serious. The report then took up the results of her investigation.

She had paid a visit to the Poole home and talked to Mrs. Poole. The Pooles had a flat in a remodeled house—living room, kitchen, bathroom, bedroom. Richard was their only child. Mrs. Poole, however, was pregnant. She was in her fifth month, often felt unwell, and spent much of her time lying down. Mr. Poole was a subway guard, and worked an early shift. He was not at home at the time of the accident. That was somewhere between eight-thirty and nine on Wednesday morning. He had been gone since six. Mrs. Poole was at home, but in bed and asleep. She didn't know when Richard had got up. He had had a slight cold for a couple of days, and she had supposed that he would sleep late, too. 'Hoped' might be a better word. Assuming, that is, that she thought about it at all. At any rate, she was mistaken. He didn't sleep late. He was up by at least half past eight. Up and about, running loose in the apartment, for all practical purposes alone. And only three years old. That was the setting. It makes a nice picture, doesn't it? Absolutely custom-built for trouble, and absolutely standard. They all begin that way.

"It was almost nine o'clock when Mrs. Poole woke up. When she finally woke up, I should say. A little earlier, around eight-thirty, she had opened her eyes for a minute, and noticed that Richard's bed was empty. Or so she decided later. At the moment, it didn't make much impression on her. She was too comfortable, too sleepy. The second time was different. She didn't just wake up—she was awakened. By a noise. It sounded like breaking glass, and came from somewhere in the flat. She rolled over and sat up, and this time there wasn't any doubt about it. Richard wasn't in his bed. She called to him, and he answered her at once and in his normal voice. He was playing in the living room. That relieved her mind, but it didn't explain the crash. She got out of bed and went to investigate. Her first stop was the bathroom, and that was it. The medicine-cabinet door was open, there was an aspirin bottle on the floor, and the basin was a litter of broken glass and vitamin pills. She stared at the mess, and then walked into the living room and asked the child what had happened. Candy, he said. He was hungry. He'd been looking for candy. In the bathroom? she said. They didn't keep candy in the bathroom. He knew that perfectly well. She told him he ought to be ashamed of himself. And so on, until he began to cry. She gave up in exasperation, went back to the bathroom, and cleaned it up. Then she put on some coffee, and returned to the bedroom to dress. She was almost dressed when it suddenly dawned on her that the aspirin bottle had been empty. Not only empty but uncapped—and no tablets on the floor or in the basin or anywhere. But it shouldn't have been empty. They had only bought it on Sunday—the day Richard caught his cold. She dug it out of the wastebasket and looked at it. It was a small bottle, but there should have been at least thirty tablets left in it.

"Miss Flynn later saw the bottle. Mrs. Poole had kept it, and showed it to her during their talk. The facts—or, rather, some of them—were on the label. It was, as expected, baby aspirin. That means colored pink for eye appeal and flavored orange for palatability. One and a half grains per tablet. There had been forty tablets in all. But, of course, no warning. Nothing about potential toxicity. Only some mumbo jumbo in fine print advising adult supervision. Nothing to frighten the customer. Nothing that frightened Mrs. Poole, anyway. At least, not at first. I don't mean that she wasn't upset. All her reactions were normal. But mostly she was simply bewildered. It was quite obvious what had happened to the rest of the aspirin pills. She realized at once. Richard had as good as told her. He'd eaten them. What she couldn't understand was why. It seemed fantastic. What had got into him? Why had he wanted to eat a bottle of pills—a bottle of medicine? It wasn't fantastic, however. Not in the least. As she learned the minute she asked him. He didn't know it was medicine. He thought it was candy.

Why? Because it tasted like candy. That was one reason. There was also another reason—just as good, or better. Mrs. Poole was like all the other mothers in our files. She had told him it was candy. She had told him so on Sunday and Monday and again on Tuesday, and probably many other times as well. It had seemed, she thought, the easiest way of getting him to take it. What Mrs. Poole did next was also painfully typical. She looked at Richard, and he looked all right. Then she asked him how he felt. He said he felt fine. I suppose she was still uneasy, but that seemed to be that. So she relaxed. It would be easy enough to blame her, but you can't. It wouldn't be fair. She didn't know that anything serious had happened. She had the universal attitude that aspirin isn't really a drug. It's something else. Because drugs are something they sell only in drugstores, and you can get a dose of aspirin anywhere— at a lunchroom or a soda fountain or on a train. It's just aspirin.

"I'm speaking for myself, of course. That's only my interpretation. Miss Flynn didn't interpret. She simply gave the facts. And one of the facts was that Mrs. Poole, understandably or not, wasn't greatly alarmed. Aspirin poisoning doesn't manifest itself in a minute. It takes a little time to catch hold. So when Richard went on playing in a perfectly normal manner, she was reassured. She calmed down. She finished dressing and helped him into his clothes, and they had breakfast. Richard didn't eat much, but there was nothing strange about that. He hadn't eaten much since Sunday. He never had much appetite with a cold. After breakfast, she got him settled with his toys in the living room, and went to work. There were the dishes to wash and the beds to make and the rest of the household chores. That must have been about ten o'clock. Well, around ten-thirty she stopped for a rest and a cigarette. Richard seemed still absorbed in his toys. She asked him how he was feeling. He didn't answer. Instead, he began to cry. She dropped down on the floor and put her arms around him, but he twisted away. That wasn't like him. He was almost never cranky. She pulled him back and felt his forehead. It was cool but wet. He was streaming with perspiration. Even his clothes were damp. After a moment, he stopped crying, and began to whine and whimper. His stomach hurt, he said. So did his head. He hurt all over. Then, all of a sudden, he vomited.

"I don't know what Mrs. Poole thought. The chances are she was too frightened to actually think. But she did what any mother would do. She picked him up and carried him in to his bed and tried to make him comfortable. Then she took his temperature. It was normal. As it always is, of course, in such cases. But it was reassuring to her, and by eleven o'clock she thought he seemed a little better. The sweating had stopped and he was resting quietly. That usually happens at about that point. Sweating and irritability are early symptoms. They soon give way to just the reverse—dryness and lethargy. Now he wasn't really resting. He was doped. In any event, he didn't seem better for long. Half an hour later, he vomited again. Then he started breathing very hard and fast—another classic symptom. That, I gathered, was when the truth began to penetrate. Hyperventilation can be a frightening sight, and it must have terrified Mrs. Poole. She couldn't call a doctor. She knew no doctor to call. The Pooles didn't have a doctor—not even an obstetrician. But I must say she kept her head. She didn't collapse or run screaming out to the neighbors. She wrapped the boy up in a blanket and took him straight to Whitestone Memorial. Also, apparently, she told them exactly what had happened. Aspirin intoxication is an extremely difficult condition to diagnose. Unless there's a clue in the history, you have to work it out by test and elimination, and even then it's very often missed. Its actual incidence is probably many times greater than any of us realize. The treatment is less complicated. It includes a prompt gastric lavage, parenteral administration of some dextrose and

93

saline solution to restore the fluid balance, and the usual supportive measures. Richard was admitted to the hospital, according to the record, at one o'clock. That meant he would have had his lavage in reasonably good time—around twelve-thirty—since they attended to that in the emergency room, on arrival. Very satisfactory.

"Well, that was the report. It told us what we needed to know, and I could assume that Miss Flynn had given Mrs. Poole some necessary instruction in the care of drugs and children. I marked it for filing and put it aside, and went on to whatever came next. As you must. Even the saddest is only one among many. By the time I got back from lunch that day, I had practically forgotten the case. And then Miss Flynn called. She had just been talking to Whitestone. Richard Poole was dead. He had died around noon. Respiratory failure. She thought I'd want to know for the record. I thanked her and hung up. I won't pretend I was more than conventionally shocked. It happens too often for that. I was, however, very considerably startled—it didn't seem in line with the facts. My impression had been that they added up to a very good chance for recovery. Thirty tablets of the size he had taken made a total of forty-five grains. Forty-five grains of aspirin is enough to cause a lot of trouble in a child of three. Anything over ten can be dangerous. As a general thing, though, it isn't fatal. I got out the report for another look. But a glance was all I needed. It was all there. It had simply slipped my mind. One of the anomalies of acetylsalicylic acid is that illness enormously intensifies its action, especially in small children, and Richard had been more or less sick since Sunday. Also, he swallowed it on an empty stomach."

The Most Delicate Thing
in the World

WE had just sat down—Harold Cousminer and I—in his gritty little first-floor office at the New York City Health Department, in lower Manhattan, when the telephone on his desk gave a shattering peal. Cousminer raised his eyebrows. "Well, here we go," he said. "But that's the way it generally is on Saturday night. Don't ask me why." He plucked the receiver from its cradle, and cleared his throat.

"Poison Control," he said. There was a pause. "Oh?" He reached for a pencil, glanced at his watch, and scribbled something on a pad of paper. "Well, I think you ought to have a gastric lavage done." He listened patiently, and nodded. "I understand, Doctor. And I agree. It's fortunate he vomited. Very fortunate. But to be on the safe side . . . You're dealing with the carbolic family, you know. That's the toxic agent there." He listened again. "O.K. Hold on a minute. I'll see what I can find." Cousminer swung around to a table at his elbow. It held a metal filing cabinet, two black leather satchels of the sort carried by doctors, a large cardboard box labeled "Calcium Gluconate for Black Widow Spiders," and a row of medical texts. He felt along the row of books, pulled out one called *The Symptoms and Treatment of Acute Poisoning*, and spread it open on the desk. After a moment, he picked up the receiver. "Hello? Well, here's the procedure—take down what you want of it. Gastric lavage as soon as posible. The choice is vegetable oil or a ten-per-cent solution of alcohol. Followed by lavage with water. Followed by demulcents such as egg albumen, egg yolk, milk, or gruel. No specific antidote. Further treatment is symptomatic and supportive. Good results have been reported from the intravenous injection of five-per-cent glucose in saline." Cousminer closed the book. "I guess that about does it," he said. "Not at all, Doctor. Glad to be of help."

"What was that?" I asked.

Cousminer shrugged. "Nothing very unusual." He leaned back in his chair. "An interne up at Roosevelt Hospital with a problem on his hands. He's got a five-year-old boy in there whose mother fed him a teaspoonful of CN disinfectant an hour or so ago. I told him what he was up against. CN is largely phenol—carbolic acid. And how to handle it, as you heard. That's what I'm here for—to answer questions like that. Primarily, anyway. A night emergency inspector also has other duties. I take complaints from the public on coal gas, carbon monoxide, and contaminated food, and when necessary I go out and investigate the situation. It all comes under the general heading of poison. But that kind of trouble accounts for only a fraction of our calls. Most of the trouble I hear about comes from toxic drugs and household chemicals. Everybody's house is full of both—especially the latter. Detergents, for example. There must be a hundred of them on the market. And deodorants, insecticides, stain removers, laundry bleaches, paints, mouthwashes, shoe polish. All plainly labeled with a big brand name and full instructions on how to use. But you very seldom see anything about ingredients—toxic or otherwise."

"Isn't there any legislation covering that?" I asked. "Something like the Pure Food and Drug Act?"

"Apparently not," Cousminer said. "I understand the American Medical Association has appointed a committee to work for a law, but those things take time. There's always a certain amount of resistance. Meanwhile, to put the matter gently, things are sometimes rather awkward for a doctor when he gets an emergency call. It can turn what might be only a minor misfortune into a real calamity. It often did until a few years ago. The idea of a clearinghouse where doctors and hospitals could get information about ingredients originated in Chicago. They established the first Poison Control Center there in 1953, and almost every large city in the United States and Canada has one now. Our center opened in the spring of 1955. The results, I'm told, have been very satisfactory. Not that there's been any decline in drug and household chemical poisoning. The average for the country is still over a hundred and fifty thousand cases a year. But there has been a drop in deaths—from upward of fifteen hundred a year to around a thousand. The reason is that the doctors don't have to work blind any more. They don't have to guess at the nature of the toxic substance in the box or bottle with the fancy label. All they have to do is step to the telephone. They know that we will probably have the answer. If the product in question is well established, the chances are it's fully discussed in one of the standard toxicological texts, and we've got them all—the best, the latest. We also have a laboratory upstairs that keeps abreast. When something new appears on the market, our chemists break it down, and the analysis goes into that filing cabinet over there. They keep an eye on the old products, too—the manufacturers change their formulas from time to time. So, one way or another, we can generally rise to the occasion. Not that we've never been stumped. We are—every now and then. But that's to be expected. You can't have a file on everything that might possibly find its way into somebody's stomach. I'm talking about accidental poisoning, of course. People don't often try to kill themselves by eating a can of Kiwi. We only hear two stories here. One is ignorance—not realizing the danger of leaving drugs or chemicals around where children can get at them. The other is carelessness. Like the case of that boy up at Roosevelt. His mother is one of the many who seem to live in a trance. She didn't notice that she was giving him CN. She thought it was his cough medicine."

"That isn't unusual?" I inquired.

"Oh, they're all unusual," Cousminer said. "It's a matter of more or less. CN seems to turn up a little more often than most. It ranks pretty close to Clorox, Zonite, and the pine deodorants. In the drug field, the chief offenders are the barbiturates and, of course, aspirin. But none of them happens every day. Or even every month. The only thing you can expect on this job is the unexpected. That's one thing I like about it. It keeps you on your toes. If it weren't for the unpredictable, the job would be hard to take—for me, anyway. The time would hang too heavy. We have a peculiar setup here, you know. It hasn't much in common with the average night-shift routine. There are five of us night inspectors, and we take our tours of duty in rotation. We work a night, lay off for four, and then come on again. But the tours we work are really tours. We start at 5 P.M., when the rest of the department goes home, and we stay with it until nine o'clock the next morning, when the day men in the various categories we combine—Environmental Sanitation, Food and Drugs, and the rest—take over. If that sounds strenuous, believe me, it is. Sixteen hours is a long time, especially at night, and in a god-forsaken part of town like this. It's endless. It's also lonely—lonely as hell —although that doesn't bother me as much as it seems to bother some of the others. I've got a few resources. In fact, the hours are mainly why I took the job. This isn't my career—I've made other plans. Which means I have to have my days and most of my evenings free. I'm thirty-two years old, I'm married, and I've got two children, but the war gave me a late start in life, and I'm still going to school." He smiled. "Graduate school at N.Y.U. I've got a master's degree in science from there, and in another two years I'll have my Ph.D. My field is geology—paleontology, to be exact. I also teach a little—I have a couple of classes at N.Y.U. and one at Cooper Union—but not quite enough to keep me afloat. I need a job, and this one perfectly fits the need. It makes the whole thing possible."

"I supposed you were a doctor," I said. "I thought you'd have to be."

"The department thinks otherwise," Cousminer said. "So does Jerome Trichter. He's the assistant commissioner who set the night-inspector service up and keeps it going. As a matter of fact, we don't need doctors on this night job. We're not here to prescribe to the general public. Our information is strictly for doctors and hospitals—"

The telephone cut Cousminer short. He sat up with a jerk, took a deep breath, and reached for the receiver. "Poison Control," he said, and paused. "I see—yes. About what time was that?" For a long moment, he was silent. He sat absorbed, gazing blindly at the wall, occasionally nodding. Then, abruptly, he said, "Oh, definitely. Very bad. Especially in a child that young. I'd say you ought to do a gastric lavage at once. But let me take a look." Opening the book he had consulted before, he found what he wanted, and frowned. He turned again to the telephone, and said, "Sorry—I was wrong. Standard procedure is Universal Antidote to start. Five or six heaping teaspoons suspended in a glass of water. *Then* lavage, with three hundred cc.s of potassium permanganate. Or an emetic—the choice is mustard or salt—to be repeated until vomiting occurs. Also, three heaping teaspoons of magnesium sulfate may be left in the stomach as a saline purgative. Acidosis is usual. It may be relieved by injecting sodium r-lactate solution intravenously until the carbon-dioxide combining power is restored, or until urine is alkaline to phenolsulfonephthalein or to litmus paper. Intravenous normal saline may be sufficient to combat mild acidosis. But I hardly think that applies in this—" He nodded. "That's right. . . . Of course—any time. . . . Absolutely. Good-by."

Cousminer pushed the telephone away. His eyes had a distant look. It was a moment before he relaxed again in his chair.

"That sounded serious," I said.

"It is," Cousminer said. "Very much so. A case of methyl-salicylate poisoning in an eight-month-old girl. Oil of wintergreen, they call it on the market. It's used as a rub for muscular aches and pains. Her parents just brought her into St. John's Hospital, in Brooklyn, which was sensible, but a little late. It happened about an hour and a half ago." He glanced at his note pad. "Around eight, the hospital said. How it happened isn't clear—except that the mother accidentally fed her a tablespoonful of the stuff. A tablespoon averages about fifteen cc.s. And six cc.s is the minimum fatal dose for children."

"You recommended something called Universal Antidote," I said. "What is that?"

"The book recommended it," Cousminer said. "I just passed it on. Although I must say I'm pretty well acquainted with it. Universal Antidote isn't actually universal, but it takes in a lot of territory. It's generally useful as a counteractive to most drugs and household chemicals. Depending on the poison, it either neutralizes the toxic agent or alters it in some way that stops or slows up its absorption until it can be eliminated. That's why it's usually followed by lavage or an emetic. The remarkable thing about it seems to be its simplicity. All it is is two parts of activated charcoal and one part each of magnesium oxide and tannic acid." The telephone rang again, Cousminer came briskly erect. "I've often wondered who thought it up," he added, and, turning, caught the receiver to his ear.

"Poison Control," he said. "Yes?" A look of incredulity crossed his face. "I'm sorry, but where did you say —" He broke off and listened. His expression cleared. "I see. Yes, of course." There was a longer pause. "Well, frankly, no. It isn't one of the big brands. But unless the label says different, it's probably acetone. Hold on, and I'll make a check." Cousminer opened *The Symptoms and Treatment of Acute Poisoning*, but after a glance at the index he pushed it aside and stood up. He moved along the table to the filing cabinet and slid out a narrow drawer. I caught a glimpse of a file of dog-eared cards, and then his shoulders blocked my view. He gave a grunt of triumph or surprise. The drawer slammed shut, and he returned to his desk and the telephone. "Hello? Well, that's the problem—acetone. Do you want the treatment? . . . That's right. An emetic—sodium chloride is preferred—or lavage. In either case, followed by stimulants to combat collapse. The choice is strong coffee, caffeine with sodium benzoate, or aromatic spirits of ammonia. If necessary, transfusion of whole blood. O.K.?" He shook his head. "Not at all. That's what we're here for."

Cousminer hung up. "Very odd," he said, and sat back, smiling. "Not the case, particularly. A six-year-old boy got hold of his mother's nail-polish remover. Fortunately, the bottle was practically empty, so he didn't get too much. Why he did it, I can't imagine. Six is a little old for that kind of foolishness. But what got me was the hospital. They took him to Lying-In. I'm surprised the staff up there had even heard of us." He smiled again, and then gave a sudden laugh. "That reminds me of a call I had one night last fall. No connections with Lying-In, of course, but also on the odd side. It was a woman—a nurse, from the sound of her voice. You can usually tell by that air of command. Was this the New York City Department of Health? I told her it was. The Poison Control Center? Yes. Were we open twenty-four hours a day seven days a week? Yes. And the telephone number— was Worth 4-3800 correct? Yes. Then she thanked me very kindly, and started to hang up. I stopped her. What was this all about? Oh, just a routine check, she said, to make sure their information was correct and up to date. Well, might I ask who was calling? Why, certainly. She thought she had told me. This was the Something-or-Other Sanitarium, in Something City, California. Apparently, they keep a list of the leading Poison Control Centers all over the country."

A heavy door slammed in the distance, and the sound of footsteps echoed down the corridor. Cousminer looked at his watch. "Coffee break," he said, and jumped to his feet. "Be back in a minute." He vanished through the door. I gazed after him into the shadowy hall, and waited. The lonely clamor of silence settled over the room. I could hear the moan of the wind in the court beyond the window. The table stretched and creaked, the wall behind me tapped, a paper stirred in the wastebasket under the desk. Overhead, the light gave a pulsating tick and seemed for a moment to dim. The room began to have a subterranean feel.

Cousminer reappeared with a lumpy paper bag. He put it on the desk, extracted two cardboard containers of coffee, and handed one to me. "Kindness of the night watchman," he said, dropping into his chair. "He remembers me when he goes out to lunch, and later on, when my time comes, I do the same for him. He answers the phone whenever I'm called out, and takes messages. Or gets someone to cover for me if a problem turns up. He's the one who let you in tonight. So he knew I had company and brought two coffees."

"Very nice," I said.

"It helps," Cousminer said, and took a long swallow.

102

He set the container on the desk. "I don't suppose you've got a cigarette?" I had, and held out the pack. Then I took one myself. "I quit smoking a couple of months ago," he said. "It gave me something to wrestle with. But now I've had my fun. I think I'll go back again."

The telephone rang. Cousminer dropped his cigarette in an ash tray and extended a hand. "Poison Control," he said. "Yes, this is the Health Department." He recovered his cigarette. "They prepared food without a permit—was that it? . . . Oh. . . . Oh, I see. Well, I'll tell you what, Call back on Monday morning and ask for the Bureau of Food and Drugs. That's the best place to file this sort of complaint." He hung up with a tolerant snort.

"What was that about?" I asked.

"Pizza pie," Cousminer said. "A member of the lunatic fringe wants us to close down a lunchroom somewhere out in Queens because they keep their pizzas in the refrigerator and heat them up on order. He's got some notion about frozen food. Thinks it's contrary to nature, I gathered. We get a good many calls like that. Outraged cranks. Drunks with a grudge. And just plain nuts. People who wake up and smell carbon monoxide—which, of course, is completely odorless, as well as colorless and tasteless. People who complain that the janitor has siphoned all the air out of their room. People who think their neighbors are trying to asphyxiate them with poisonous incense. They'd almost be funny if they weren't so sad."

Cousminer stubbed out his cigarette and sat back with his coffee. "I remember one call I got about a year ago," he said. "I'll never forget it. A woman over in Brooklyn. Said her apartment was full of fumes. She'd been smelling them all evening—this was around 2 A.M.—and they were getting stronger and stronger. It was all she could do to breathe. I asked her to describe the odor, but it seemed she couldn't. Nobody could, she said. It was indescribable —oh, too revolting for words. Well, I wasn't much impressed by that. It had a fairly fishy sound. On the other hand, she was obviously sober. No more excited than you'd reasonably expect. Gave me her name and address in a very businesslike way. So I said O.K., I'd be right out. You can't take chances on anything involving gases or fumes. You have to go and see. Which I did. It was a run-down building in a run-down neighborhood—a Chinese laundry on the first floor, a roaring saloon across the street, and a used-car lot on the corner. A perfect environment for trouble. And when I got upstairs and she opened the door, I was sure of it. She was just as sensible-looking as she sounded. I put her down for a retired schoolteacher—around sixty-five, and as neat as a pin. So was her apartment. I went through it room by room. No odors, not a sign of gas—nothing. I don't mean I just thought so. I knew it for a fact. We don't guess or estimate on a gas investigation. We use instruments. Our equipment includes an explosimeter, to see whether the gas content of the air is near the exploding point; a manometer, for measuring gas pressure; and a CO meter, which will detect even the faintest concentration of carbon monoxide. Along with various tools. They're all in that satchel over there on the table—the fat one. The other bag is Food and Drugs paraphernalia. Bottles and cartons for samples. Embargo forms. Et cetera. Well, it took me about an hour. I even went down in the cellar and poked around the furnace. She had me that convinced. But finally I was satisfied, and I told her so. She gave me a look that curled my hair. Did I mean to say I couldn't smell the fumes? That's when I first saw the light. I didn't say no. Instead, I asked where they seemed to be coming from. No answer. Just another look. Then she took me by the arm and marched me over to the front window and pointed across the street—at the saloon. Now could I smell it? I obliged her by sniffing, but that wasn't enough. I had to say something. I asked her what it was she smelled. 'The odor of rotting souls,' she said."

Cousminer drank off the last of his coffee. He crushed the empty container and pitched it into the wastebasket. "Maybe she did," he said.

"I wouldn't know," I said.

"No," he said. "Neither would I. I've got a speculative turn of mind. At least, I like to use my head. But not in that direction. I suppose that's why I'm a paleontologist, and a night inspector. The problems that interest me—and the kind I usually get—are a little more down to earth. I don't care how tricky they are. All I ask is that when you finally put two and two together, the answer turns out to be four. Not x. I've had some tricky ones, too. I remember one not long ago that gave me a certain amount of mental exercise. As a matter of fact, I can think of two. The first was another Brooklyn case, and it also involved a saloon. That's where the story began. The scene had changed, however, by the time I came into the picture. My introduction was a telephone call from King's County Hospital—a doctor in the emergency room, with the usual request for help. Only it wasn't exactly usual. It was a case of vegetable poisoning. The victim was a Puerto Rican, a man about thirty, and the history he gave the doctor was this: He had dropped into a bar on his way home from work. After a couple of drinks, he got to talking with the bartender, and somehow the conversation got around to a big decorative plant in the window. It had been there for years, the bartender said, but he had never known what it was. The Puerto Rican said it looked like sugar cane. Another drink and he was certain. To prove his point, he broke off a piece of the stalk and started chewing it the way they did when he was a boy back home. The next thing he knew, his mouth was on fire. Then his throat. He had never felt such pain. Then his face began to swell, and he realized what had happened—he'd been poisoned. So he headed for the nearest hospital. By the time the doctor saw him, his face was so swollen he was hardly able to talk. Examination showed a violent

105

inflammation throughout the mucous membrane of the mouth, tongue, and throat, and he was very obviously in agony. He was also, it seemed quite clear to the doctor, in very serious trouble. But what kind of trouble? What was the plant? What was its toxic principle? And what, if any, was the antidote or treatment?

"I told the doctor I'd see what I could do, and call him back. Not, however, with much enthusiasm. It looked hopeless. To be frank, I didn't even know how to begin. There wasn't much point in searching the files or trying one of the texts we have on poisonous plants. You can't look something up unless you know its name. The only possibility I could think of at the moment was Harry Raybin. Raybin is technical director of the center and one of the men we can call on for help in an emergency. Another, of course, is Mr. Trichter, but his field is primarily environmental sanitation. So I put in a call for Raybin, and got him at his home. That's all, though. He was as stumped as I was. Which left me with a choice between Trichter and a needle-in-the-haystack hunt through Muenscher's *Poisonous Plants*. But before I could make up my mind, one of those nice things happened. I had an idea—a hunch. I called the Bronx Botanical Garden. It was after hours and the office was closed, but eventually somebody answered. A watchman, and very obliging. When I hung up, I had the names and telephone numbers of all their top botanists. As it turned out, one was enough. Or perhaps I simply picked the right man first. Anyway, I told him the story and he told me the answer. It was as simple as that, and almost as quick. It sounded, he said, like *Dieffenbachia seguine*. Sometimes known as dumb cane, and indigenous to tropical America. In fact, it couldn't be anything else. Moreover, he added, I could rest assured that there was nothing to worry about. *Dieffenbachia* was not a poisonous plant. It took me a minute to absorb that piece of information. Then I reminded him that, after all, the man was in the hospital. In a great deal of pain. Swollen up like a pumpkin. Only just able to speak. No doubt, he said, but that was not the result of chemical damage. It was purely mechanical, and essentially harmless. One of the characteristics of *Dieffenbachia* was its secretion of very sharp crystals of calcium oxalate. And one of the consequences of chewing the plant was temporary loss of voice. That's why it was called dumb cane."

Cousminer smiled a fleeting smile. I had left my cigarettes on the desk, and he helped himself to one. "The other case I mentioned was less exotic," he said. "And quite a bit grimmer. It started, for me, with a police report. That was one evening last January. I'd just come on duty when they phoned it in. A couple of hours before, the superintendent of a tenement over on East Broadway had found one of his tenants—a bachelor around thirty-five or forty—dead in bed. I've forgotten how he made the discovery, but that part isn't important. He did, and called the police, and they came up, and one look was all they needed. No question about the cause of death. The man was sprawled on his back in a very untidy tangle of bedclothes, and his face was cherry-red. A classic picture of carbon monoxide. The medical examiner placed the time of death at about 7 A.M., and said there was good reason to believe that the man was an alcoholic, or at least a heavy drinker. Well, those were the facts, except for one thing. It wasn't suicide. There were no gas outlets open. That made it an accident, and a case for us. So I got my bag of tools and went over to East Broadway. It turned out to be a three-story building of cold-water railroad flats, built about 1910, and in fair repair. The dead man's apartment was top floor rear, but my first stop was the super's—on the floor below—for the keys and anything else that might be useful. He told me the man had lived there for years, originally with his parents. They were both dead now. His father

had died two years before, and his mother just the previous month. Since her death, the son hadn't spent much
time at home. Had all his meals out, and only rolled in
to sleep. The apartment confirmed that much. It was the
usual three-room layout, with the kitchen in the middle,
and a lot of gas equipment—refrigerator, kitchen range,
and two or three space heaters. But, as the police had
found, they were all turned off or out of use. The refrigerator was even disconnected. However, none of the
things were in very good shape. For all I knew, they were
leaking at every joint. I unloaded and went to work. I
spent an hour or more on the fittings alone. Then I covered every inch of the place with the CO meter. But no
soap. I didn't find anything that might even hint at
trouble. The apartment was safe, and, that being the
case, my job was done.

"This was around seven-thirty. I remember looking at
my watch when I finished packing my bag. Then, all of
a sudden, I smelled smoke—coal smoke. It came from
the kitchen, and by the time I got there, it was already
good and thick—too thick for comfort. The source was
plain enough. It was seeping out of an unused stovepipe
vent that was capped with an old pie tin on the wall above
the gas range. But why? How come the smoke wasn't
going on up the flue? I opened a window to clear the air,
and decided I'd better find out. There was a ladder at
the end of the hall that led through a hatch to the roof.
I climbed up and out, and went over to the chimney. It
was letting off smoke, but not much—just a little wisp. I
flashed my light down the flue, and you never saw such a
rat's nest. Sticks, old rags—all kinds of trash. I don't know
who did it—kids, probably—but it was a very thorough
job and, from the look of the junk, one that had been
going on for quite some time. Well, that explained the
smoke in the dead man's kitchen, and maybe a whole lot
more. Coal smoke is an excellent source of carbon monoxide. At any rate, I had to locate the fire, if only to put

it out. The super's apartment seemed the place to start. One reason, of course, was its location, directly below the dead man's rooms. But I really think the super's help was all I had in mind at first. Until he opened the door. Then I caught a whiff of burning coal. I followed my nose to the kitchen, and there it was—a potbellied stove, going to beat the band. The rest, after I'd put out the fire, took about three minutes. I learned that the super only used the stove to take the chill off his flat. His usual time was now, in the early evening. But sometimes he used it for an hour or two in the early morning. That morning, he recalled, had been one of those times. I didn't need any more. When I added that to what I already knew about the dead man's habits, the picture was in focus. The tenant came home and fell into bed. Let's say around midnight or so. A few hours later, the place began to fill with smoke, but he was too drunk to wake up, and slept right through to eternity." Cousminer shrugged. "That's my theory, anyway."

"It sounds very reasonable to me," I said.

"It fits the facts," Cousminer said. "I've also got another theory. Or maybe suspicion would be a better word. On the way back here, I got to thinking about the dead man's parents. I wondered if there might be some connection between their deaths and his. Particularly his mother. It was simply curiosity, but I wanted to know. Several days later, I dropped in at the Bureau of Records and Statistics here in the Health Department and had a look at their death certificates. They made rather interesting reading. I don't mean I found any proof—none whatever. But the cause of death in both was something that could have been brought about by a dose of carbon monoxide."

The telephone rang. Cousminer discarded his cigarette and took up the receiver. "Poison Control," he said. "That's right." He listened, and frowned. "I'm afraid I don't follow you. . . . Yes, I got that—it's spelled D-e-l up to where the label's torn. But what's it supposed to be used for? There must be some hint on the bottle. I mean—" He nodded attentively. "I see. Clear as mud. However—hold on while I check our file." He rose and went over to the cabinet and pulled out a drawer. After a moment, he slammed it shut, and walked thoughtfully back to the phone. "Sorry," he said. "We've got nothing of that description in the files. Must be something very new. But, judging from what you say, it's almost certainly a solvent. Which would probably make it benzine or one of the chlorinated hydrocarbons. . . . Oh? It does, eh? Well, if it smells like benzine . . ." He reached for *The Symptoms and Treatment of Acute Poisoning* and heaved it open. "O.K. The thing to do is empty the stomach by lavage. Saline solution. And that's it. Not much else you can do in the way of emergency treatment. . . . Yes, I hope so, too. Good night."

Cousminer sat for a moment gazing at his notes. Then he shook himself and slumped back in his chair. "Well, that's one way to build up the file," he said. "I can think of better ones, though."

"What happened?" I asked.

"A two-year-old out in Manhasset got hold of what sounds like some sort of benzine preparation," he said. "I gather it's used for cleaning radio parts—'to restore volume control and contact' is the way the label puts it. That's about all I know, except that she just arrived at the North Shore Hospital, and her chances are pretty slim. Nonexistent, I should imagine. According to the doctor, she swallowed about two ounces of the stuff."

"Oh," I said.

Cousminer gave me a curious look. "Yes," he said. "Very sad." He hesitated. "That's the standard reaction, isn't it? But somehow I've never felt that way. I don't mean that I'm hardhearted. Or hardboiled—like a Belle-vue interne. And I'm certainly not indifferent. It's just that my viewpoint is a little out of the ordinary. I told you I was in the war. I was a gunner on a B-24, and I flew thirty-five missions. That experience was part of it. The rest is what I've seen on this job, and what I've learned as a paleontologist. Most people take life for granted. My feeling is that it's not that dependable. In fact, it's the most delicate thing in the world. It's a miracle. And one false step and it's over."

Ten Feet Tall

OF all the wonderfully mettlesome drugs that crowd the contemporary medicine chest, two distinct but functionally related substances, called cortisone and ACTH, are by far the most vivacious. They are also the most peculiar, the most provocative, and the most dimly understood. Neither, in the usual sense, is a therapeutic agent. Unlike the sulfonamides, the antibiotics, and even, perhaps, the vitamins, they possess no curative powers. Though often spectacularly brilliant, their salubrious effects, which include the relief of pain, the reduction of fever, and the reversal of crippling infirmities, are seldom more than palliative and almost never permanent. In this respect, they resemble nothing so much as aspirin. The resemblance is not, however, otherwise pronounced.

Cortisone and ACTH are hormones. A hormone is a chemical mediator produced by the body and essential to maintaining its intricate equilibrium. The term derives from *hormao*, the Greek word for "excite," or "stimulate." The manufacture of hormones is among the several functions of the several ductless glands—the thyroid, the parathyroid, the pituitary, the adrenals, the gonads, the thymus, and the pancreatic islets of Langerhans—that form the endocrine system. Since 1902, when the British physiologists Sir William Bayliss and Ernest Starling first demonstrated the role of an endocrine secretion in the

112

digestive process, some twenty different hormones have been identified and studied. Their range of influence has yet to be fully established, but it is known to embrace such factors as body size, mental tone, metabolic tempo, and sexual development and capacity. Around ten of these substances, including ACTH (or, more formally, adrenocorticotropic hormone), are pituitary products. The pituitary is both the smallest and the most important of the ductless glands. By the sporadic release into the blood stream of one or another of its numerous hormones, each of which stimulates a specific gland, it regulates the hormonal output of all the other endocrines. ACTH stimulates the cortex of the adrenals. This is a barklike layer of tissue that elaborates, among other hormones, one known to biochemists as 17-hydroxycorticosterone, from which another, called 17-hydroxy-11-dehydrocorticosterone, can be derived; 17-hydroxy-11-dehydrocorticosterone is cortisone.

The development of cortisone and ACTH, like most scientific triumphs, was the work of several variously gifted hands. Cortisone came first. Its discovery was charted in 1930, when investigators at Princeton, Ohio State University, and elsewhere demonstrated for the first time that adrenal cortical extracts prepared from animal glands possessed definite hormone powers. Five years later, it was isolated, also from animal glands, by Tadeus Reichstein, a professor of organic chemistry at the University of Basel, and Edward C. Kendall, a biochemist on the staff of the Mayo Foundation for Medical Education and Research. A test devised shortly therafter by a Mayo physiologist showed it to be biologically active. ACTH was isolated in 1943. A biochemist named Choh Hao Li and some colleagues of his at the University of California are among those prominently associated with its discovery. A team of Armour & Company chemists, working with pig pituitaries, managed to produce a small amount of ACTH in 1946, but several more years passed before it was available in even experimental quantities. By then, cortisone had been mastered. In 1948, after six years of hard labor, Lewis H. Sarett, a chemist in the employ of Merck & Company, evolved a synthesis that made it possible to produce cortisone commercially. It was given its first clinical trial by Philip S. Hench, chief rheumatologist at the Mayo Clinic, in September of that year. The results were all but dumbfounding.

Hench, like many others, had for some time suspected that there might be a connection between adrenal insufficiency and rheumatic disease. He therefore chose for his pioneering test a victim of rheumatoid arthritis. The patient was a woman of twenty-nine, bedridden and in almost constant misery. Hench placed her on a course of a hundred milligrams of cortisone a day. After only three days of treatment, she was able to move without pain. The next day, she felt even better, and it was possible for her to stand unaided and take a few halting steps. Four days later, she walked out of the clinic for an afternoon of shopping. She returned, after three hours, no more than normally fatigued. Hench halved her dosage, and hoped. Nothing happened. Reassured, he reduced it again by half. For several days, the patient continued to move about freely and comfortably. Then, little by little, the familiar symptoms reappeared, and by the end of a week, she was locked once more in agony. Hench put her back on a hundred milligrams a day. Her decline abruptly halted, and again she began to improve. Hench and his associates (Kendall, C. H. Slocumb, and H. F. Polley) sat down and reviewed the experience. Its meaning seemed reasonably plain. Six months later, having repeated the test, with identical results, on thirteen more arthritics, it was clear beyond any question. Cortisone (and, as Hench was subsequently inspired to discover, ACTH) had an incomparable capacity to relax the grip of one of man's cruelest diseases. It also, most certainly, provided medical science with an investigative tool of truly inestimable value. But it was not a cure. It was, for all its extraordinary energy, only an alleviative.

The usefulness of cortisone—and what is said of cortisone may generally be said of ACTH—is not confined to rheumatoid arthritis. Since April, 1949, when Hench announced his galvanic find (in the pages of *Proceedings of the Staff Meetings of the Mayo Clinic*), medical journals throughout the world have rung with testimonials by other clinicians to its efficacy in other ailments. The number of diseases upon which it has been reported to have at least some analgesic impact now approached the galaxial. They include acute iritis, Addison's disease, asthma, choroiditis, Cushing's syndrome, dermatomyositis, erythroblastosis fetalis, gout, hay fever, Hodgkin's disease, lumpus erythematosus, lymphatic leukemia, myasthenia gravis, pemphigus, periarteritis nodosa, ivy poisoning, retinitis pigmentosa, rheumatic fever, scleroderma, spondylitis, Still's disease, tetanus, ulcerative colitis, uveitis, vernal conjunctivitis, and Waterhouse-Friderichsen syndrome. It has also been found to be helpful in the treatment of shock, burns, and fractures. It has even been seen, among victims of alopecia totalis —a baldness of possibly metabolic origin—to stimulate the regrowth of hair.

Dazzled by this evidence of vigor and versatility, many investigators have come to consider cortisone almost a panacea. So, even more enthusiastically, have many more physicians. There is, however, in both these groups a core of stubborn dissenters. Their opposition to the popular view is only distantly rooted in doubt. It is prompted chiefly by discretion. They do not question the potency of cortisone. What they question is its safety. Hormone therapy, they point out, is still largely an empirical science. Just how cortisone achieves its impressive results has yet to be adequately explained. They therefore feel that until its mechanisms are more clearly illuminated, and the nature of its long-range, or cumulative, effects determined, the general use of so formidable a substance is more than a little rash. Their prudence is understandable enough. There is, at the moment, no reason whatever to assume that the long-range effects of cortisone are benign. There is some reason to suppose them pernicious. Even its immediate effects, though usually of limited duration, are not always wholly admirable. They can be most unpleasant. In fact, the violence and variety of the toxic reactions that may be induced by cortisone render it—again, together with ACTH—unique among drugs. Some of its side effects are those of any occasionally toxic drug (nausea, headache, skin eruptions), and others, as might be expected, are the familiar grotesqueries of endocrine imbalance (gross obesity, moonface, hypertension, diabetes, softening of the bones, development of facial hair in women and children), but as many more are new—awesomely new. A common consequence of hormone therapy is lowered resistance to infection. The presence of cortisone in the body creates an environment that seems to be warmly hospitable to most known pathogenic microorganisms. Among the microbes whose proliferation it demonstrably encourages are streptococci, staphylococci, pneumococci, brucellae, typhoid bacilli, spirochetes, and the viruses of influenza, Coxsackie disease, and poliomyelitis. (Its effect on the tuberculosis bacilli, in particular, appears to be practically tonic.) It has the power to revive a vanquished infection, it can excite a latent one to manifest itself, and, in the opinion of some investigators, it may even be capable of transforming into antagonists certain normally innocuous viruses. It can also unhinge the mind. Mental derangements unequivocally attributable to cortisone have been reported by hundreds of clinicians. In many cases, these disturbances simulate with absolute fidelity the syndromes classically characteristic of paranoia, schizophrenia, and manic-depressive psychosis. "It is difficult to be sanguine about drugs with such side effects as these," Lewis Thomas, head of the pathology department at the New York University-Bellevue Medical Center noted in a recent study, "and it is not enough to say that some of the reactions are transitory or reversible, or that they do not occur very often. If these can be the immediate effects, we should await the much later effects of treatment, especially prolonged treatment, with meticulous attention, and, I submit, with some anxiety." To this, Henry J. L. Marriott, professor of medicine at the University of Maryland, has added, "We are dabbling in the unknown with dangerously potent tools."

The ugly side of cortisone does not, of course, completely contraindicate its use. It merely suggests its reservation for crises of intolerable pain or peril. Even the wariest clinicians concede that cortisone has a place, and a triumphant one, in modern chemotherapy. The relief it can bring to the racked and hobbled victims of rheumatoid arthritis would alone compel its inclusion. There are several other, though less prominent, diseases against which it is even more providentially effective. One of these, as a New York City schoolteacher I'll call Robert Laurence can readily testify, is periarteritis nodosa. Were it not for cortisone—and ACTH—Laurence would now be either bedfast and dying or dead, for until the advent of hormone therapy, periarteritis nodosa, a destructive inflammation of the arteries, was almost always briskly fatal. His escape was accomplished, however, at a truly hair-raising price.

Laurence teaches history and English at a day school for boys. He is married and has a son of eleven and lives in a frame and stucco house in the Forest Hills section of Queens. He is a robust man of medium height, with brown eyes and a sandy crew cut, and he had just turned thirty-eight when he became acquainted with cortisone. That was on the morning of January 23, 1954, in a hospital I'll call Whitestone Memorial. He had then been sick for more than a month and in the hospital for almost a week, but the nature of his trouble had finally been firmly established only the day before. Even at that, he was lucky. Periarteritis nodosa, though reasonably easy to diagnose if suspected, so closely resembles so many more common diseases that it not infrequently eludes recognition right up to the autopsy table. He was also fortunate in his immediate reaction to cortisone. The amount prescribed by his doctor—Prince, I'll call him—was a hundred and fifty milligrams a day, and the effects of this treatment were prompt, positive, and wholesome. Within a week, Laurence was up and about, restlessly prowling the ward, all symptoms and signs of inflammation vanished. His disease, if not uprooted, had at least been checked and was now safely under control. On Monday, February 1, he was found fit to resume a normal life, and discharged.

Despite his exhilarating recovery, Laurence went home from the hospital no more than mildly elated. His mood reflected his valedictory interview with Dr. Prince. The physician opened the meeting with a word of congratulation, moved on to a round of reassurances, and closed it with instructions to call at his office for a progress review the following Monday evening. Meanwhile, he added, producing a prescription, he was increasing the daily dose of cortisone to an even two hundred milligrams. "That was a little disturbing," Laurence says. "It made me wonder. If I was coming along as well as he said, why did I need more cortisone? Why weren't a hundred and fifty milligrams still enough? But I kept my doubts to myself. Some doctors will tell you the reason for every move they make. Dr. Prince is one of the others. He believes in a minimum of explanation and a maximum of results. And, of course, I said nothing to my wife. Nora isn't easily upset, but she and Bobby were so happy and excited to have me home again, I couldn't. I wouldn't have anyway. It wasn't that important. There was only one important thing. The only thing that really mattered was being out of the hospital and back home—and well. I knew I was well. Nobody had to tell me that. I hadn't felt so good in years. I don't mean just physically. It was more than that. I felt as bright as a button—capable of anything. It was really extraordinary. It was almost as though I'd never been fully awake before.

"We were between semesters the week I came out of the hospital. That gave me time to get caught up and ready for work again. The spring term opened on Monday, February 8. I don't know when I've had a better opening day. I never felt better, and I never got my classes organized and functioning more efficiently. My mind was like some wonderful precision instrument. Everything I did was right, and absolutely effortless. I remember driving home from school that afternoon and marveling. I felt as fresh as when I'd sat down to breakfast. It was just as well I did. I found my wife in bed. She'd been fighting the flu for a couple of days and had finally given in. I got a chair and sat by the bed, and we talked for a while—mostly about dinner and the household chores. Then Bobby came in from playing, and when he came upstairs, he brought the afternoon paper. I picked it up and started turning the pages, and all of a sudden an advertisement caught my eye. It was a picture of a dress at Best & Company. The price was thirty-five dollars, but it was a beauty. It was black jersey and very plain—just the sort of thing Nora looks wonderful in. I showed it to her and she thought so, too. It was lovely, she said. The rest is hard to explain. I mean now. At the time, it seemed perfectly natural. It was only what any intelligent man would do. We have a telephone extension in the bedroom, on my night table. I looked up the number and called the store and they had the dress in Nora's size. I told them to send it out."

Mrs. Laurence's attitude toward this act of impulse has also been altered by time. Its meaning now is painfully clear to her. It then seemed merely peculiar. "Bob has always been interested in clothes," she says. "He likes me to dress well and he has very good taste. So there was nothing strange about his interest in that ad. But we had hardly reached the point where he was selecting my clothes for me. And we weren't exactly in the habit of buying thirty-five-dollar dresses sight unseen. Why, I've known Bob to spend half an hour just picking out a shirt. He's terribly particular. On the other hand, it did look like a really darling dress. I didn't know what to think—except, of course, that if it wasn't right, I could always send it back. Besides, I guess, I wasn't really able to think. I had one of those headaches that leave you simply limp. The oddest part, though, wasn't *what* he did. It was how he did it—his manner. He was so terribly polite to the people at the store. And so talkative. I thought he'd never hang up. And when he did, it was almost worse. He jumped to his feet and came around to my side of the bed and started talking a mile a minute. It was something about people wasting all their time on trifles. I tried to listen and pay attention, but I just couldn't. I felt too sick and miserable. He went on and on. Finally, something he said seemed to remind him that he was the cook that night. He looked at his watch and said he'd better get started or he'd be late for his appointment with Dr. Prince.

"I remember hearing Bob go down the stairs. He called to Bobby and they went into the kitchen, and I lay there and listened to them talking and moving around. Then I must have dozed. The next thing I knew, Bob was standing by the bed with my dinner on a tray. Bob is quite a good cook and it was a lovely dinner—cold roast lamb, mashed potatoes, string beans, salad, hot biscuits, some kind of pudding, and coffee. But, good heavens! Food was about the last thing in the world I wanted. Particularly that kind. So I said so. It never occurred to me that Bob wouldn't understand. Well, he practically jumped down my throat. Nonsense, he said. I had to eat. Everybody had to eat. How did I expect to keep up my strength if I didn't eat? But I wasn't hungry, I said. It would make me sick. 'Don't be silly,' he said. 'Eat your dinner.' It was fantastic, but I was simply too baffled to argue. I managed to swallow a few bites. Then I had an idea. I asked him to get me something—I've forgotten what—and while he was out of the room, I scraped the rest of the food into part of the paper and bundled it up and hid it under the covers. It seems so ridiculous now, so childish—and also so sad. Because it worked. Bob took the tray away without a single question. He was perfectly satisfied. And so was I. In spite of everything, all I really felt was relief. My only problem was staying awake until Bob left for his appointment. As soon as he did, I slipped downstairs and dumped the evidence in the garbage can. Then I crawled back to bed.

"I didn't hear Bob come in. He was already in bed, with the lights out and the window open, before I even knew he was home. What woke me up was his fidgeting. He was so nervous and restless it was actually shaking the bed, and every bounce made my bones ache. It was agony. I asked him what in the world was the matter. Nothing, he said. He just couldn't get comfortable. But the moment I heard his voice, I knew better. He was frantic with worry. Sick as I was, it frightened me. I'd almost forgotten that he was the one who was really ill. I had to know the truth, and I insisted until he told me. It was the doctor. Dr. Prince had increased his cortisone —for the second time, I learned. The dose was now two hundred and fifty milligrams a day. This time, Bob had insisted on finding out why. Bob was doing fine, the doctor said, but it was important at this stage to make certain that the inflammation remained completely smothered. I think that's how he put it. Also, I believe, it had something to do with determining Bob's maximum tolerance to cortisone. I suppose I *was* a little surprised at the increase. However, I couldn't see that it was anything to get alarmed about. As a matter of fact, the reasons that Dr. Prince had given sounded very sensible to me. But they didn't to Bob. More cortisone simply meant that he wasn't getting well. The doctor was only trying to humor him. He was probably getting worse. And so on. I've never seen him so frightened—not even at the very beginning of his illness. I remember wondering if that might explain the way he'd been acting earlier. It was possible. Anxiety can make people do very strange things. Anyway, I did the best I could to reassure him, and he calmed down a little. He kept tossing and turning, though, and finally I suggested that he spend the rest of the night in the guest room. I thought he might sleep better in a bed by himself. He didn't want to, but I was firm. I was sure it was the best thing under the circumstances. In the end, he went, and I fell asleep. I don't know how long I slept. It seemed to me I had just dropped off when I heard my name. It was Bob. He was bending over me, and he was crying. I mean literally. There were tears rolling down his cheeks. He didn't like it in the guest room. It was too lonesome. He missed me and needed me. Wouldn't I please let him stay? It was pathetic. I couldn't bear to see him so upset. So I said all right. What else could I do?

"It was nearly eleven o'clock when I woke up the next morning. That isn't like me, even when I'm sick, so I must have been utterly exhausted. Bob and Bobby, of course, had both left long ago. I wasn't feeling quite so wretched, and after the night before, I wasn't sorry to be alone. It gave me a chance to rest in peace. The first one home was Bob. Bobby has a music lesson after school on Tuesday. Bob had hardly been out of my mind all day, and I didn't know what to expect. I dreaded another scene. Well, I've seldom been more startled. He bounced into the room like Fred Astaire. He had his biggest pipe in the corner of his mouth and the afternoon paper under his arm, and he couldn't have looked less worried. Last night might never have happened. It seemed to have vanished from his mind. I just lay there and stared. Everything he said was a joke. He was absolutely bursting with high spirits. When he leaned down for a kiss, he gave me a hug that almost broke my back. But he was as restless as ever. He perched on the bed. Then he moved over to a chair. A minute later, right in the middle of a sentence, he jumped up and started pacing. Then I must have closed my eyes for a moment. Suddenly, he let out a kind of hurrah. He was standing on the far side of the bed with the paper in his hand. It was folded open to one of the inside pages, and he held it up for me to see. 'Listen to this!' he said, and started reading. But he didn't have to tell me. I caught a glimpse of B. ALTMAN and MEN'S SUITS and TWENTY PER CENT OFF, and that was enough. My heart sank. I watched him pick up the phone and dial the number. It was just like the day before. Except he was even more polite. It took him forever to get to the point. But when he finally did, he couldn't have been more businesslike. Single-breasted gray flannel. Size 40. Charge and send. There was a pause. Well, what *did* they have in his size that was nice? He frowned. He didn't think he'd ever seen a brown slash weave. He nodded. But didn't the red and green make it rather loud? No? Then send it out. And while they were at it, if they saw anything else that might appeal to him—another suit, or maybe a topcoat—send that along, too. I just lay there and stared. I was speechless. It wasn't that I begrudged him a new suit, or even a topcoat. But, good heavens—what in the world had come over him!

"But Bob was completely oblivious. He hung up with a flourish and came striding around the bed. He lighted his pipe and rubbed his hands and cleared his throat. He asked me if I realized the significance of what he had just done. It wasn't a question, though. He went right on. An important principle was involved, he said, and it illuminated a whole philosophy. Our life lacked order, and we needed a new sense of proportion. We had become incapable of distinguishing between the important and the trivial. Our one most vital possession was time, and we squandered it like drunken sailors. When it was necessary to buy something—a dress, a suit, a piece of furniture—we thought nothing of running into Manhattan and spending an entire afternoon traipsing from store to store. It was shocking to think of the hours we wasted every year so foolishly, and so needlessly. But no more. From now on, we would do things differently. He waved a hand in the direction of the telephone. There was the answer. We were privileged to live in a day of instant communication. It was high time we took advantage of it. He felt that the experiment he had conducted this afternoon sufficiently proved his point. It was possible for an intelligent man to select—comfortably, easily, and at a substantial saving—a fine suit of clothes in a mere matter of minutes. Perhaps I questioned his use of the word 'select'? That was an interesting point. His choice had, of course, been guided by the clerk. But it was equally true that a store of Altman's age and reputation would hardly employ an incompetent man. The man quite obviously knew his job. He had taste and integrity. We were too often inclined to be cynical. Most people were basically fine and decent and trustworthy. We must have confidence in our fellow man. We must learn faith. We must realize that whatever happens is usually for the best. Then he went back to the beginning. It was shameful for intelligent people to waste themselves on trifles. There were more important things in life than clothes.

"Bob must have talked for a solid hour. He probably wouldn't have stopped even then if Bobby hadn't come in and asked about dinner. It's hard to remember now just what I thought at that stage. Everything changed so completely after that. Dinner was only an interlude. It was another huge meal and I still felt much too wretched to eat, but it wasn't as bad as the night before. At least there was no one standing over me. Bobby brought up my tray. I didn't see Bob again until after dinner—until after he'd done the dishes, in fact. He walked in and sat down and kicked off his shoes, and I remember thinking that he seemed almost relaxed. Bobby was watching television, he said. As for himself, he was going to take a bath. I reminded him that he had just washed the dishes and there wouldn't be much hot water left. He'd better wait a little while and give the boiler a chance to recover. He smiled, and said that wasn't the point. He wanted to take a bath. He wanted to take it now. Was it my impression that he was the kind of man who could be dictated to by a machine? If there was no hot water, he would bathe in cold. I said I hardly thought that the middle of February was the best time for a cold bath. He gave me a surprised look. No? Why not? Water was water. Temperature was a mere detail. It meant nothing. It did in his condition, I said. A cold bath might do him a great deal of harm. If he must bathe now, I said, I'd get up and go downstairs and heat some water on the stove. I never dreamed he'd let me. But he simply shrugged and said all right, go ahead. For a moment, I just felt numb. And then I knew. I couldn't avoid it any longer. I'd been able to rationalize the dress and the suit and the tears and the wild, crazy talk. But this was different. This wasn't Bob. There was no resemblance whatever. This was a man I'd never seen before. Something had happened to Bob—something terrible. I let him help me out of bed and stand me on my feet, and then I went tottering down the stairs. He didn't even offer to come with me."

Laurence has no clear recollection of that tyrannical bath. He only remembers having a sense of power and glory. Exaltation had become his natural state. Every impulse seemed to quicken it. On Wednesday, driving home from school, he passed a plumbing and heating establishment. The cogs of memory and acquisitiveness meshed. He pulled up and went in, and ordered a new capacious, rapid-recovery hot-water heater and boiler. "I knew I'd done an extraordinary thing," he says. "And yet it seemed so right. So sensible and necessary. So exhilarating. All my instincts confirmed it. I came out of the shop in a glow. I was tingling. But that night, in bed, an awful feeling came over me. Had I been right? It may have started with the way Nora looked when I told her what I'd done, but it went deeper than that. It was basic. Everything seemed suddenly hopeless and empty and wrong. It only lasted a minute, though. I shook it off the way you sometimes can a nightmare. Of course I'd been right—everything I did was right. I'd felt so sure of it before. I was more than right. I was supreme.

"I lay awake a long time after that. I was too excited to sleep. When I finally did drop off, I hardly slept at all, and I was wide-awake before it was even light. But I felt completely rested. I was bursting with strength and energy. It was as though I'd reached a new level of existence. Sleep didn't seem to matter any more. A few minutes was as good as an hour. My only real necessity was food. I'd had a tremendous appetite all week, but Thursday morning it was almost frightening. There just wasn't any limit to my capacity. I had a tumbler of orange juice, a bowl of oatmeal, a big plate of scrambled eggs, five or six pieces of toast and jelly, and I don't know how many cups of coffee. It wasn't nearly enough. My stomach was like some bottomless pit. I put away two more big bowls of oatmeal before I really felt comfortable. Then I was ready for anything. By the time I got to school, I was keyed to concert pitch. I seemed to be on the verge of something enormous. Something wonderful was going to happen. The feeling kept building up all morning, until there wasn't any doubt about it. I was sure. My first class after lunch that day was a class in English composition. We were just settling down to work when one of the boys slid out of his seat and started toward the door. That wasn't in the least irregular in our school. The pupils don't have to ask to go to the washroom. But a kind of thrill ran through me. I let him reach the door, and then, very quietly, I spoke his name. 'May I inquire where you are going?' I said. The boy was stunned. It was all he could do to answer. 'I see,' I said. 'Well, I suggest that you return to your seat. If you wish to leave the room, you will do me the courtesy of asking my permission.' He still looked stunned, but he managed to get back to his seat and mumble something acceptable. I excused him with a friendly nod. When the door closed, I turned back to the rest of the class, and it was like a revelation. In an instant, my whole conception of the student-teacher relationship was altered. The teacher was more than a purveyor of academic instruction. He must also set an example in character and command. The evidence was written on every face in the room. It was as plain as print. I had won their respect and admiration. Boys wanted discipline. It was a fundamental need in adolescence. They weren't prepared for freedom of action and self-expression. It only confused them. They longed to conform. They wanted rules and regulations and, above all, firm direction. But the discipline that fully answered their need was not, I realized, the discipline of common coinage. They wanted a humanistic discipline—strict, but administered with understanding and affection. It seemed incredible that I had never seen the truth before. We no longer were forced to choose between the old schoolmaster system of teaching and the new progressive method. I had found a middle way.

"There was a faculty meeting after school that afternoon. It was like an act of fate. I was bursting to share my discovery with my colleagues. Just before we adjourned, I asked permission to say a few words. I began with a brief account of the washroom incident. Then, as simply as possible, I described the principle of humanistic discipline. I felt, I went on to say, that it should be adopted by the school. It was imperative that we make every effort to respond to the emotional needs of our students. Anything less was irresponsibility. I talked for about ten minutes. When I finished, the director rose and thanked me, but there was no discussion. The other teachers just sat there looking thoughtful. They looked almost bewitched. But as the meeting broke up one of my best friends took me aside. He suggested I take it easy. There was a good deal of truth in what I said, he told me, but I was a trifle unrealistic. Changes must be accomplished slowly. I heard him out, and smiled. It was a pitying smile. "I'm sorry to hear you talk like that,' I said. 'You really shock me a little. I had no idea that you were such a cynic.' I gazed at him for a moment, and it was pathetic. He looked so insignificant. He seemed to have shriveled up to nothing. Then I turned and walked away. I felt ten feet tall."

Laurence was not alone in this alpine impression of himself. It soon was shared by both his wife and his son. "Thursday was my first day out of bed, so I was still working when Bob got home," Mrs. Laurence says. "I was cleaning the living room. Everything had gone to pieces while I was sick. I heard the car in the drive and his steps on the porch, and then the door opened. It flew open. I remember looking up, and—I don't know how to explain it. It was the queerest feeling I ever had. He looked enormous. He really did look ten feet tall. Bobby said the same thing later on. He seemed to fill the room. It was his manner, I think, and the way he held himself. And his voice. That was part of it. The instant he saw me, he started talking, and I've never heard such colossal self-assurance. Such conviction. It was something about something at the school. A new era was about to dawn. He had discovered a new technique that would revolutionize the present methods of teaching. It would revolutionize the whole of American education. He stood on the threshold of a new career. His life was no longer aimless. He had a mission. I did my best to listen and pay attention. It made a kind of sense at times. Only he talked so fast. He was almost incoherent. The words simply poured out. After about ten minutes of just standing there, I picked up my things and very quietly went on with my work. He didn't seem to notice. He was too excited. All I had to do was nod when he looked at me. He stormed up and down the room, and his ideas got wilder and wilder. The new technique didn't only apply to teaching. It also applied to domestic life. Our home was to be run on the same basis. The keynote was discipline. He loved me, he said. He bounded over and threw his arms around me. And he loved Bobby. He loved us both with all his heart. But he was our leader. He was in command. From now on, our home would be run on a basis of strict paternal control. There would be no more preoccupation with trifles. The day of laxity and foolishness had passed. Discipline was the new order. He followed me into the dining room. Did I understand? He pounded on the table. There had to be discipline. It was the only way to happiness. Then, all of a sudden, he stopped. It was as if he had just run down. He walked into the living room and picked up his coat and hat. He was going out, he said. The house was too small for him. He needed air, and room to turn around in.

"Well, I was limp. I sat down and tried to think. By then, of course, I did have a kind of inkling. I wasn't quite as mystified as I had been a day or two before. I was pretty sure I remembered reading or hearing somewhere that sometimes cortisone had strange effects on people. If so, it must be that. There wasn't any other explanation. I couldn't believe that Bob had actually lost his mind. But that wasn't really much help. It didn't tell me what to do. My brain went around and around and around. I finally told myself that this was pointless. Dr. Prince knew what he was doing. He was a specialist —one of the best. The sensible thing to do was keep busy and try not to worry. Everything would be all right. I got up and finished cleaning the dining room, and then went out to the kitchen. It was still too early to start dinner. So I decided to do some ironing. I'd done a long-overdue washing that morning, and I knew that Bob was down to practically his last shirt. I set up the ironing board and connected the iron and went down in the basement and picked out a couple of his favorites. As I started back up, I heard somebody in the kitchen. I thought it was Bobby, but it wasn't. It was Bob. He was standing in the middle of the room with the iron in his hand, and he was livid. He turned on me like a tiger. Just what did I think I was doing? Hadn't he made it clear that there would be no more preoccupation with trifles in this family? Did I think he would permit his wife to drudge her life away at an ironing board? I was not a menial. I was his wife, and he expected me to conduct myself as such. He slammed down the iron. I was to get all this paraphernalia out of his sight at once. Immediately. Did I hear?

"I told him I heard. But he had to have clean shirts, I said. He couldn't go around in a soiled shirt. The look he gave me was absolutely withering. He had no intention of wearing a soiled shirt, he said. There were such things as laundries. He supposed I had heard of them. I said all right. I agreed with him. But I tried to be reasonable. I suggested that at least I go ahead and iron the shirts that I had already washed. After all, I said, he had to have something to wear while the rest were at the laundry. That was as far as I got. He blew up. He began to yell that he wouldn't live like this. He refused to complicate his life with all these petty problems. He didn't give a hoot about laundries or anything else. He couldn't be bothered. From now on, he'd buy a new shirt every morning and throw it away at night. Life was going to be simple in this house or, by George, he would know the reason why. That was the law. I didn't wait for any more. His face was beet-red and he was shaking like a leaf. I disconnected the iron and folded up the ironing board and put them back in the closet. I wasn't humoring him. It wasn't like Tuesday night. He meant exactly what he said. It was an order."

Friday was Lincoln's birthday, and a school holiday. Nevertheless, Laurence again rose early, and, after another hearty breakfast, drove over to the school. He thought he felt like catching up on his work. That impulse, however, quickly petered out. He was too restless to concentrate on anything for long. At the end of an hour, he gave up, and decided to get a haircut. The shop he chose was a two-chair place near his home, and it was jammed. "There must have been eight people ahead of me," he says. "But I wasn't in the least annoyed. Quite the contrary. I was delighted. Company was just what I wanted. I'd hardly said a word all morning. And it turned out to be delightful. I don't know when I've spent two more completely enjoyable hours. One of the customers was a man who lived a few doors from us. He knew I'd been sick, and he was nice enough to ask me how I was feeling. I sat down and told him all about it, and he seemed very much interested. He never took his eyes off me. So I went on to tell him some of my views on current events. My interpretation of the news also seemed to interest him. It seemed to interest everybody in the shop. Even the barbers were listening. That was very exciting and stimulating—up to a point, anyway. But then I began to wonder. A sort of suspicion edged into my mind that I might be making myself a little conspicuous. So I put on the brakes. I tried to keep my voice down and take it easy. When my neighbor was called to the chair, I even looked at a magazine for a while. Then

I got up and just wandered around. By the time the barber was ready for me, I'd made friends with everybody. They couldn't have been more pleasant. They seemed to hang on every word I said. I'd never realized before how easy it was to mold people to my will. It was as though they were just waiting to be told what to think and do. I had a sense of rapport with everybody in the world.

"Except Nora. Just before I left the shop, I took the trouble to call her up. I wanted her to know where I was and that I would be home soon and not to worry. We only talked for a minute, but I hung up in a foul humor. It wasn't anything she said. She was exactly as she always is—sweet and natural and matter-of-fact. It was more her attitude. She wasn't like the others. We weren't in tune. She didn't respond. The whole point of my call escaped her. She didn't seem to realize what a thoughtful thing I'd done—how kind and considerate I was to put her mind at ease. She simply accepted it. It was infuriating. It practically ruined the morning. But that wasn't enough. I had hardly walked into the house when she did it again. Another letdown. On the way back to the car, I passed a little haberdashery shop, and a necktie in the window caught my eye. I went in and bought it, and it was really beautiful. It was made of some rich material like brocade. Well, I showed it to Nora and she agreed with me. She was enthusiastic. But it was flawed, she said, and pointed out a streak across the front where several threads had slipped. She thought I ought to exchange it. I tried to control myself, but it was too much. It was like a slap in the face. Apparently, everything I said went in one ear and out the other. After all our talks, she was still wrapped up in trifles. It seemed incredible that anyone could be so obtuse. I can't remember what I said. Maybe I don't want to. The next thing I remember is running up the stairs. I almost felt like laughing. It was so ironic. There was only one woman in the world I could love, and I'd outgrown her. I ran into the bedroom and slammed the door behind me. It didn't matter. None of it mattered. I threw myself on the bed and started kicking my feet and pounding the pillow. I began to yell how wonderful I felt. I yelled how happy I was. Then, all of a sudden, I wasn't yelling any more. I couldn't. I was crying."

It was a little past noon when Laurence bolted up to the bedroom. He remained there—mostly, after the first outburst, in an obviously misanthropic silence—for the better part of an hour. At one, Mrs. Laurence heard him open the door and come slowly back downstairs. "I was in the kitchen with Bobby," she says. "I remember we looked at each other and exchanged what was supposed to be a reassuring smile. Bobby had missed most of that awful scene in the living room—he was playing next door, thank heaven. But he'd heard enough. He'd come in just in time to hear Bob shouting and yelling, and nothing could have been more unnerving than that. I'd tried to make him understand, of course, and I think I did, but even so—He looked so tense I almost wanted to cry. I could have cried for Bob, too. He seemed so oblivious. He strolled in without a word and drew himself a glass of water and swallowed his one-o'clock cortisone. Right on the dot. It was as if nothing whatever had happened. Then he came over and asked if we weren't going to have any lunch. I could hardly believe my ears. To think that after what had just happened he still felt like eating. But I fixed something, and we all sat down. It was incredible how he ate. His appetite was bigger than ever. The only time he even paused was to snap at Bobby and me for just picking at our food. When he had finally had enough, he jumped up and marched out. He was going for a walk. That must have been around two. A little before three, he came charging back—bursting. We were going to trade in our Plymouth on a brand-new Studebaker. I was paralyzed. I couldn't say yes to something we didn't need and couldn't afford, and I was afraid to say no. The clock saved me. I reminded him that he was due at the store in less than half an hour. Bob has a part-time job. A friend of ours owns a bookstore over on Queens Boulevard, and Bob helps him out on Friday afternoon and evening and all day Saturday. He enjoys it, and it gives us a chance to buy books at a very attractive discount. We could discuss a new car later, I said. As it happened, we never did.

"I spent the rest of the afternoon catching up on my work. After dinner, Bobby helped me with the dishes, and then we played a game of Scrabble. We were looking at television when Bob got home. For a minute, it was just like any Friday night. He called hello the way he always does and hung up his coat and hat and started toward the sofa. I thought he was going to sit down beside me. I think he meant to. But he didn't. He suddenly stopped dead in his tracks. He was staring at the television set as though he had never seen it before in his life. So this was how his family spent their time, he said. His voice was like ice. We had a house full of books. We had a phonograph and a library of the world's greatest music. But, apparently, we were just like all the rest of the country. We preferred *My Friend Irma*. Was that our intellectual level? He gave a howl that almost froze my blood. No wonder we couldn't keep pace with him. No wonder we couldn't give him the sympathy and understanding he needed. No wonder he was all alone. He let out another yell, and dived across the room and shut the program off. Then he backed away a step and doubled up his fist. Maybe this would bring us to our senses. He'd show us what he thought of television. He was going to take his fist and smash that screen to pieces. He would have, too. It wasn't just a threat. But Bobby moved first. He slid out of his chair and ran over to the desk and pulled open the drawer where we keep the telephone book. Bob heard him, and whirled around.

And what was he up to? Bobby was white as death, but he told him. He said he was looking up Dr. Prince's number. He thought he ought to be here. Indeed, Bob said. He pointed his finger at the sofa. Bobby had exactly one second to get over there and sit down and be quiet. He wasn't to move a muscle. Neither was I. We were to sit there and nothing else, no matter what. No matter what he did. He might put his fist through that screen. He might decide to kick the whole set apart. He might even take a knife and cut off one of his fingers and throw it in the wastebasket. But we were to just sit there. Was that clear?

"I don't know what came over me. It wasn't courage. I was still completely terrified, but something had broken the spell. It must have been seeing Bobby try to call the doctor. Whatever it was, it gave me the strength to get to my feet and tell Bob what I thought. I told him this had gone on long enough. We knew he was sick, but that was no excuse. I wouldn't stand for it. Besides, it was almost eleven o'clock. Bobby should have been in bed an hour ago, and I refused to keep him up another minute. Bob didn't say a word. He just looked startled. I moved fast. It was either that or collapse. I spoke to Bobby and caught his hand, and we were out of the room and up the stairs before Bob could even blink. He must have been absolutely stunned. While Bobby was getting undressed, I stood at the door and listened. There wasn't a sound. He was still downstairs, and that gave me an idea. We couldn't go on like this. I had to talk to the doctor, and now was my chance. I got Bobby settled and calm enough to close his eyes and relax, and then I slipped down the hall to our bedroom. But I'd waited too long, or maybe Bob heard me. Our bedroom is right above the living room. I had only dialed the number when I heard him racing up the stairs. The next thing I heard was Dr. Prince's voice. By some miracle, he answered the phone himself. I managed to say hello and give him my name. Then Bob was there and reached over my shoulder, and broke the connection. His face was like stone. I wanted to run. All my brand-new bravery was gone. He replaced the receiver and leaned against the wall and looked at me. I supposed he was trying to decide what to do. For one horrible moment, it crossed my mind that it might not be me he was thinking about at all. It might be Bobby. And then the phone rang. I looked at Bob. He sort of shrugged. I waited, but that was all. So I picked up the receiver and said hello. It was Dr. Prince. We seemed to have been cut off, he said. He added that I had sounded a bit disturbed. Was something wrong? I said yes. I didn't dare say any more than that. He hoped Bob wasn't sick? I said no, not exactly—and prayed that he would understand. He did—in a way. So that was it, he said. Not acting like himself, eh? I said yes. Talking too much? Easily excited? Moody? I said yes. Well, cortisone could do that, he said. Especially in the amount that Bob had been getting. It was nothing to worry about, of course, but still— Suppose I brought him in tomorrow for a check. He could miss a day at the store. It would probably do him good. I said I'd try to. Meanwhile, Dr. Prince said, if I had such a thing as a sedative, that would calm him down very nicely. I said I thought we had some Luminal. Fine, he said. Just the thing—and hung up. I could have screamed.

"I won't go into the next four hours. They were a living nightmare. Bob stormed all over the place. He raged and ranted. He cried. At one point, he even took a bath. He apologized a thousand times. I was terrified. I was furious. I would have run out of the house and left him, if it hadn't been for Bobby. We ended up at four o'clock in the bedroom. That's when he finally agreed to take the Luminal. There was only one capsule in the bottle, and he had been trying his best for half an hour to knock it out of my hand. He didn't want to go to sleep, he said. He was never going to sleep again. Sleep was a waste of time. Then he got the idea I was trying to poison him. He didn't trust me, he said, and if I didn't leave him alone, he would tear off his clothes and run out in the street naked. That was one threat. I've forgotten the others. But at last he gave in. I brought him a glass of water, and he took the capsule and put it in his mouth. He kept it there just long enough for me to relax. Then he reared back, and spat it clear across the room. I remember scrambling after it. I was practically hysterical, but I knew it was the only hope I had. I had to find it. And I did. I found it, damp and dirty, under the bureau, and brought it back. I was so wild I must have frightened him. He swallowed it—dirt and all.

"Bob's appointment with Dr. Prince was for two o'clock Saturday afternoon. It was obvious that he wasn't eager to go, but he went. I think he remembered enough about the night before to realize that he had behaved very badly. During the drive downtown, he hardly said a word. He seemed completely subdued. But I knew that mood too well. I wasn't deceived, and I prayed that Dr. Prince wouldn't be. It didn't seem to me he was, but it was hard to tell. He asked Bob some questions about his general condition and he made some tests, and that was about all. There were only two encouraging things. One was just after we sat down. He asked Bob how he was feeling. Bob closed his eyes and smiled. 'I'm as contented as a contented cow,' he said. That was fine, Dr. Prince said, but he glanced at me and sort of frowned. The other thing was really two. He gave Bob half a grain of phenobarbital and an envelope of phenobarbital capsules. He was to take one every three or four hours until further notice. And he reduced his cortisone from two hundred and fifty to a hundred and fifty milligrams. Bob left the office still pretty much subdued. We got in the car and started home, and he began to tell me how sorry he was about last night. He was ashamed of himself. He didn't know what had come over him. It wouldn't happen again. I sat and listened. I was almost tempted to believe him.

"We were almost home when he suddenly let out a yell. He jammed on the brakes and started pounding the wheel. I was the one who ought to be ashamed, he said. I never thought of anybody but myself. Maybe I thought he hadn't noticed, but he had. He'd seen me yawn just then. He understood everything now. I didn't care what happened to him. I was too self-centered. The car behind us started blowing its horn. People were turning around and craning their necks and grinning. It was so awful I wanted to die. I begged him to be sensible. I told him it wasn't true. I said I hadn't yawned or, if I had, it didn't mean what he thought. I wasn't any of those things. I did sympathize. I did care. He must know that. And after an eternity, he began to calm down a little. He stopped shouting and put his hands back on the wheel, and we drove on. But only a couple of blocks. When we came to the neighborhood shopping center where I do most of my marketing, he swung over to the curb and parked. I asked him what this meant. He said it was Saturday. Didn't I have some week-end marketing to do? It was true. There were several things I needed, but he had such a strange look on his face that I didn't know whether I dared leave him. He might do anything. He might even go home without me—and Bobby was there alone. But I had no choice. He opened my door and practically pushed me out. So I went. I've never gone through an A. & P. so fast. In spite of Saturday afternoon, I was back in less than fifteen minutes. And Bob was still there. He was standing beside the car, watching me. I began to breathe again. He took the groceries and stowed them away and I started to get in. There was a package on my side of the seat. It was wrapped in gray and white striped paper and tied with red ribbon. Bob was beaming like a boy. He told me to open it up. I did, and inside were a couple of handkerchiefs from a specialty shop across the street, and a card. It read, 'To my Valentine.' I looked at Bob. For an instant, there was something about him that puzzled me. Then I realized what. He looked life size. He looked like Bob again."

But he wasn't—not quite. Mrs. Laurence was, understandably, mistaken. She was not, however, mistaken about Dr. Prince. He hadn't been deceived by Laurence's professed serenity. He had recognized that his patient was suffering from a cortisone-induced manic-depressive psychosis, and he acted with reasonable dispatch. The following afternoon, Laurence was readmitted to the hospital, and the program of cortisone treatment was suspended. He remained there this time for a week. On Wednesday morning, he requested a pen and some paper from a nurse, and in thirty minutes jotted down a record of his experiences, as he recalled them, during the past three weeks.

"I do not fully realize yet how toned up I was and still am," he wrote, in part. "Although I have been off the drug since last Sunday—today is Wednesday, February 17, 1954—there is still evidence of strange, yet wonderful things. I find that when I begin to talk, I talk incessantly. On Sunday, as soon as I got in bed, a complete sense of well-being overcame me. I developed complete and utter faith in the doctor and in the hospital staff. I feel a kind of floating sensation. Physically, I seem strong beyond imagination. For the first three days, I experienced an insatiable hunger—as though I could eat a hundred meals at each serving—and yet I was able to control the urge to eat. Now I am able to wait for meals and do not seem to be hungry between meals. Mentally, I am as sharp as the proverbial tack. On Tuesday and today, I demonstrated to doctors, nurses, and other patients some remarkable feats. Crossword puzzles, which I usually left unfinished during my previous stay at the hospital after thirty to forty minues of patient effort, fall victim to my mind in five minutes. I completed today's cryptogram in the morning newspaper, which I had never had enough patience to even begin in the past, in about one half hour. Mathematically, I find I can multiply two numbers in my head, such as 84 times 36, and get the product, 3024, almost as quickly as it takes me to write about it. Early yesterday afternoon, one of the patients showed me a page in her French reader. I read as fluently as if I were a native of France. Of course, elementary French is easy and I have always been able to read it fluently, but in recent years there have been moments of stumbling over words which seem to be absent today. Relative to the very writing of this account, it has been years since the words flowed so smoothly and the pen wrote so unhaltingly. Emotionally, I still exhibit a tendency to become annoyed by the petty behavior of the people around me, but now I can exercise remarkable control where strangers are concerned. I am even beginning to think that my overt behavior with most people is altogether normal. But with my wife, there remains a desire to impress upon her the rightness of my views, to mold her and to change her until she conforms completely to the artificial pattern I am setting up for her. I know it's wrong, and at present it seems to be the major part of the battle. I must reinstitute the controls which I have always exercised. I must realize that her behavior is not constituted of faults but that my standards of the past few days are out of line. Finally, I know nothing about medicine and I cannot discern what the doctor sees when he is examining me, but I appear to be healing. In fact, as crazy as it may seem, there are times when I seem to *feel* the healing process."

On Sunday, February 21, at Dr. Prince's suggestion, Laurence was released from the hospital for a spell of rest at home. About three weeks later, on March 12, some symptoms of periarteritis nodosa having reappeared, his doctor ordered him back to the hospital for what turned out to be a stay of about a month. Hormone therapy was resumed on a trial-and-error basis, and this led to the substitution of ACTH for cortisone. By the time Laurence was discharged from the hospital, forty units of ACTH, taken every four days, had been established as the optimum course. That was on April 10, 1954. He has been comfortably free ever since of any symptoms of either periarteritis nodosa or manic-depressive psychosis.

You will also want to read
these adventure stories by
GERALD DURRELL

X910 *THREE TICKETS TO ADVENTURE* (60c)

"Adventure" was the name of a tiny village near the mouth of the Essequibo River in British Guiana. In this book, the author starts off on another of his wonderful and exciting quests for live specimens of animals for the zoos of the world.

X923 *THE DRUNKEN FOREST* (60c)

In the "drunken" forest—a remote section of Uruguay, where the borracho trees bear a wine-jar appearance—you will meet Eggbert the bird, who made the author literally laugh until he cried; terrible toads; the four-eyed birds; the tired anaconda; and many others ...

X944 *A ZOO IN MY LUGGAGE* (60c)

The story of Durrell's travels in West Africa to assemble his own stock of rare creatures, for his personal zoo ... "(he) proves to have his novelist brother's ability to impale the butterfly of reality on the point of a pen."—TIME Magazine

X956 *THE WHISPERING LAND* (60c)

The scene this time is lower Patagonia, and "the layman will find this book a delight, with never a dull moment from Buenos Aires to Patagonia, thanks to Mr. Durrell's extraordinary ability to communicate his exuberant pleasure in his chosen work."—New York Times

You will also want to read

FOLKSING (S1062—75c)
Edited by Herbert Haufrecht

A big, rich collection of over 150 folk songs from many times and many lands. Here is a panorama of America in song—sad songs and stirring ones, romantic songs and funny ones—songs of the sea, of heroes, villains, of cow-punchers and lovers false and true—work songs, game songs, calypsos, spirituals, Gay '90's songs—and ballads old and new.

The collection includes many favorites which cannot be found in similar anthologies, and provides complete words, music, guitar chords and extra lyric sheets for community folksings.

MEMORIES OF A CATHOLIC GIRLHOOD
by Mary McCarthy (S1211—75c)

The author of THE GROUP has written one of the most unusual autobiographies of the century. Miss McCarthy's vivid memories of an unusual childhood recreate a delightfully warm, sensitive, yet witty portrait of a young girl who became, according to *Time*, "quite possibly the cleverest writer the U. S. has ever produced."

These books available at your local newsstand, or send price indicated plus 10¢ per copy to cover mailing costs to Berkley Publishing Corp., 15 East 26th Street, New York, N. Y. 10010